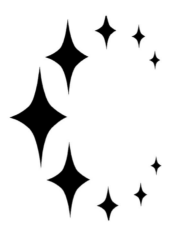

CONSTELLATION
PUBLISHING LLC

Please note the following important cautions before using this book. Not all exercises are suitable for everyone, and this or any exercise program may result in injury. Consult with your doctor before embarking on this or any other exercise program. The creators, producers, performers, participants and distributors of this product cannot guarantee that this program is safe and proper for every individual. For that reason this program is sold without warranties or guarantees of any kind. Any liability, loss or damage in connection with any use of this program, including but not limited to any liability, loss or damage resulting from the performance of the exercises demonstrated here, or the advice and information given here, is expressly disclaimed.

Hints: Practice this program on an empty stomach or at least 2 hours after eating a meal. Practice on a non skid sur-face. Never force yourself into a posture longer than it feels comfortable for you.

CONTENTS

4 INTRO LETTER TO YOU

Welcome to a new level of yoga!

6 BENEFITS OF CHAIR YOGA

Some of what you'll experience when incorporating a yoga practice.

8 STARTING YOUR PRACTICE

Before you begin lets talk about breath and posture.

THE MOVEMENTS

Before you start the postures, these movements are your starting point.

14 - 43 UPPER BODY

44 - 57 CORE AND MORE

58 - 85 LOWER BODY

ROUTINES TO TRY

Start your day, end your day, or focus on a specific area of the body.

88   MORNING STRETCH

This gentle morning stretch will help increase flexibility & mobility, improve circulation and reduce stress!

90   10 MIN. TOTAL BODY STRETCH

Rejuvenate from head to toe with this total body stretch!

92   AB FOCUSED ROUTINE

These core focused moves engage and challenge multiple muscles in different ways, leading to a more functional core.

94   HIP & BACK RELIEF

Create more mobility, release tension and reduce pain in your hips and lower back.

96   STRENGTH ROUTINE

Tone and strengthen with this quick but very beneficial yoga routine.

98   UPPER BODY TENSION RELIEF

Relax and refresh with this gentle routine, releasing tension in your upper body while improving range of motion in your joints.

100 BEDTIME RELAXATION ROUTINE

Release tension and clear your mind with this gentle yoga practice.

WELCOME TO A WHOLE NEW LEVEL OF YOGA

CHAIR YOGA IS ADVANCED YOGA

I say this because you're not only receiving the benefits of a gentle yoga practice, but you're able to relax more into each pose as your body is fully supported by the chair. This beginner friendly form of yoga is the perfect entry point into a practice. It can even be more effective than a traditional yoga practice especially if you're struggling with balance and stability, knee or back pain, mobility issues, recovering from an injury or surgery, or unable to get up and down off the ground.

This *Beginners Guide to Chair Yoga* is not only the perfect place to start, but can also be used to resurrect a yoga practice that you may have given up on or felt you could no longer keep up due to the demands of a traditional yoga practice.

There's a myriad of ways yoga helps to enhance your quality of life, and it's been my mission to help make yoga accessible to as many people with different physical abilities as possible. I have been teaching accessible yoga, using a chair for support, for the last ten years including through our PBS TV program, "Happy Yoga with Sarah Starr." It is a great honor to share this gentle, supportive and extremely beneficial practice with all of you.

No matter where you are in your journey with yoga, this guide is suitable for all ages, body types and fitness levels and will help give you the basics of integrating a chair yoga practice into your daily exercise routine.

Yoga, by definition, is the union of mind, body, and breath. Chair yoga is all of that and more while using a chair for support... It's that simple.

In keeping simplicity in mind, I'm excited to help you get started on your chair yoga journey.

- With Love and Support for your Journey,

Sarah

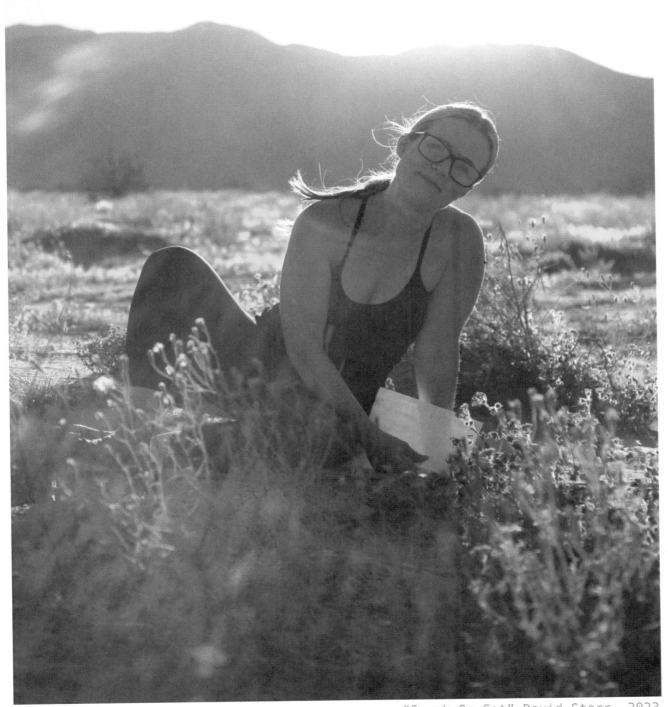

"Sarah On Set" David Starr, 2023

BENEFITS OF CHAIR YOGA

Some of the benefits you will experience when you practice chair yoga include:

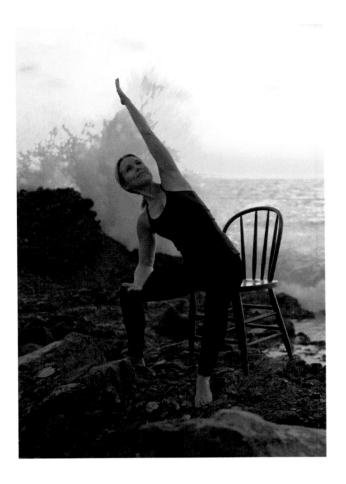

1. Improved flexibility and range of motion in your hips, spine, and shoulders.

2. Increased flexibility and strength in the muscles of your arms, legs, and feet.

3. Reduced joint pain and stiffness, which is especially helpful if you have arthritis or other chronic conditions that affect your joints.

4. Improved posture by strengthening the muscles that support your spine.

5. Improved balance and coordination which help reduce the risk of falls and other accidents.

6. Improved circulation which can help reduce the risks of heart disease and diabetes.

7. Reduced stress and improved mental clarity through the use of mindful breathing and relaxation techniques.

CHOOSING AND PO-SITIONING YOUR CHAIR

Things to keep in mind when choosing your chair:

1. If possible, use a chair that does not have sides.

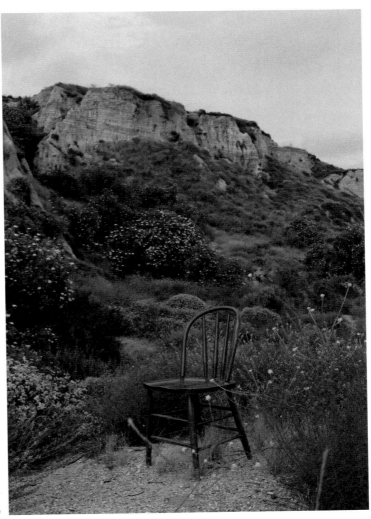

2. Make sure your chair is the right height for your body type. It's beneficial to sit in a chair where your feet are flat on the ground with your thighs parallel to the earth. Depending on your height, you can use yoga blocks under your feet to bring your thighs parallel or sit on a blanket or cushion if you have longer legs.

4. For more stability and security, it can also be helpful to place your chair on a carpet or a yoga mat.

3. If your chair has wheels, make sure it is positioned securely and the wheels are locked.

POSTURE

Many yoga practices start with focusing on your breath, but before we do that, let's begin with our posture.

———————

Maintaining good posture is important while practicing chair yoga and for general overall health and well-being. Good posture helps to prevent pain and injury by keeping your bones and joints in proper alignment. It also helps you to improve your breathing habits, allowing you to expand your lungs fully to take deeper breaths. Good posture helps you to distribute your weight evenly across your body, improving balance and stability. It also reduces fatigue and increases your energy by helping to reduce stress on your muscles and joints. Lastly, it helps to improve your appearance, allowing you to look more poised and confident.

Here are some tips for maintaining good posture while seated in a chair:

1. Sit up straight in your chair with your feet flat on the ground.

2. Keep your spine straight, with your shoulders down and back and your chest lifted.

3. Avoid slouching or rounding your shoulders.

4. Keep the back of your neck long with your head in line with your spine and over your shoulders.

5. Keep your shoulders over your hips and your hips grounded in place.

6. Place your feet hip-width apart, with your knees over your ankles and your thighs parallel to the ground.

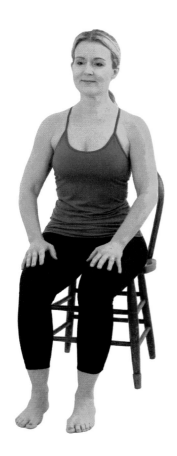

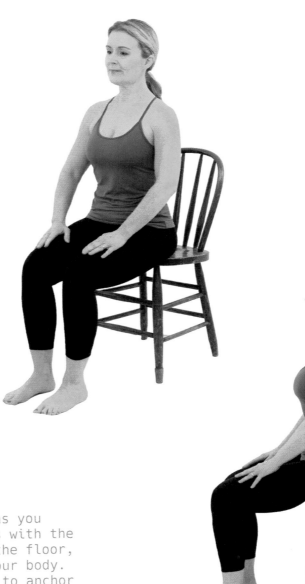

It's important to pay attention to your posture throughout your chair yoga practice. Take time to adjust your position as needed to maintain good alignment and comfort.

Notice the sensations as you feel the contact points with the chair, the support of the floor, and the alignment of your body. Engage all your senses to anchor yourself in the present moment and deepen your awareness.

THE BREATH

Belly Breath

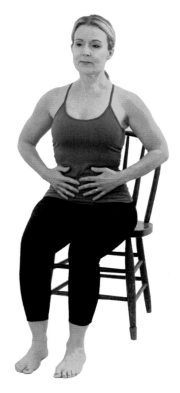

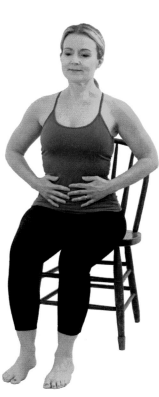

Put yourself in a comfortable position, and place your hands on your belly, at the space below your navel.

1. Inhale slowly and deeply. You will feel your belly expand like a balloon and your navel move away from your spine.

2. On your exhale, feel your navel draw back towards your spine. Exhale fully.

3. Inhale easily. Feel your belly expand again.

4. Exhale fully, and feel your navel draw back towards your spine.

5. Continue for as long as you like. This is the natural way of breathing, like a baby's breath.

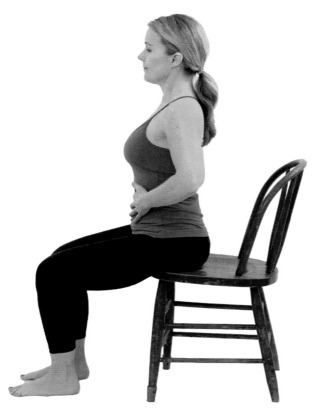

Use your breath as an anchor to keep your attention directly in the present moment. Notice the sensation of the breath as you inhale and exhale during each pose.

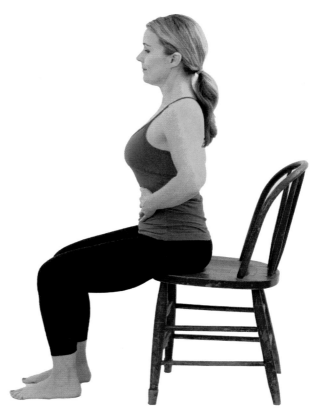

THREE PART BREATH

The three part breathing exercise is a simple yet powerful breathing technique. It can help calm the mind and body and also help improve focus and concentration.

1. Sit in a comfortable position with your back straight and your feet firmly on the ground.

2. Place both hands on your belly. Begin by taking a deep breath in through your nose. Allow your belly to expand as you inhale. Next, exhale slowly through your nose. Allow your belly to contract and draw your navel back towards your spine.

3. Place your right hand over your right rib cage. Inhale from your belly to your ribs. Exhale belly, then ribs.

4. Place your left hand over your heart. Inhale belly, ribs and chest, feeling your chest expand and rise. Exhale belly, ribs and chest.

Continue to breathe in this way, focusing on the three parts of the breath. As you breathe, try to maintain a slow and steady rhythm, and focus on the sensation of the breath moving through your body.

Continue to practice this breath for several minutes, or for as long as you like.

The three part breathing practice can help improve the quality of your breath, promoting deeper relaxation and a sense of calm. Practice this breathing technique regularly and use it as a tool for managing stress and anxiety.

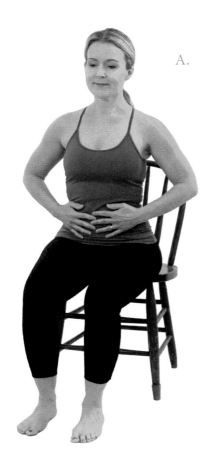

A.

If possible, try to continue using this breath throughout your yoga practice.

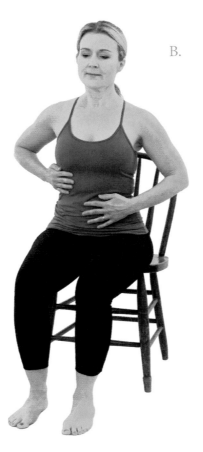

B.

C.

Stay present and keep your attention fully engaged in the current pose or movement. Avoid getting caught up in thoughts about the past or future. If your mind wanders, gently bring your focus back to your breath and the present moment.

SHOULDER SHRUGS

This exercise helps to improve the flexibility and strength of your shoulder muscles, while reducing tension and stiffness in your upper back and neck.

1. Sit up straight in your chair with your feet flat on the ground and hip width apart. Your arms should be relaxed.

2. Slowly lift your shoulders up towards your ears. Hold this position for a few seconds, then slowly release and return to the starting position.

3. Inhale lift, exhale to release. Repeat the movement several times, lifting and releasing your shoulders slowly and smoothly.

4. Continue coordinating this movement with your breath. Inhale lift, exhale lower, noticing how your exhalations begin to ease away any tension.

*Avoid tensing up your neck or
upper back muscles, and focus on
keeping your arms relaxed.*

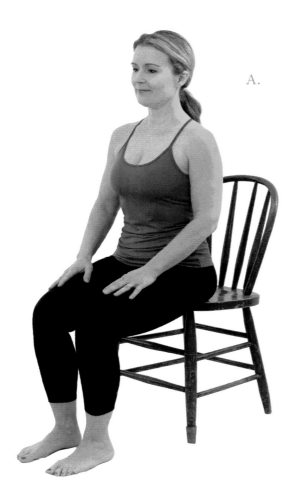

A.

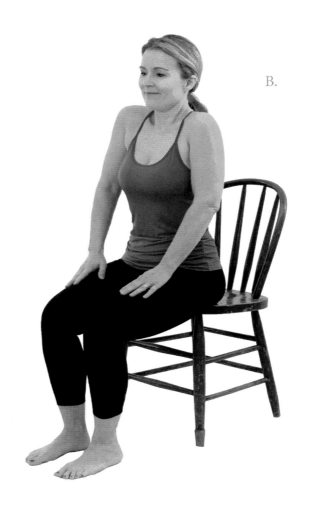

B.

Practice moving at a slower pace,
allowing yourself to fully experience
each movement and transition. Avoid
rushing through poses and instead
savor the sensations and awareness
that arise.

NECK ROTATIONS

This movement helps to reduce tension and stiffness in your neck while improving flexibility and range of motion.

1. Sit up straight in your chair with your feet flat on the ground and hip width apart. Your shoulders should be down and back.

2. Slowly turn your head to the right, looking over your shoulder as far as you comfortably can. Hold this position for a few seconds, then slowly return to the starting position.

3. Inhale at center, and exhale while repeating the same movement to the left side.

4. Keeping your spine straight and your neck long, continue moving from right to left, allowing this movement to originate from the point between your shoulder blades .

5. Repeat 10x on each side, gradually increasing your range of motion with each exhale.

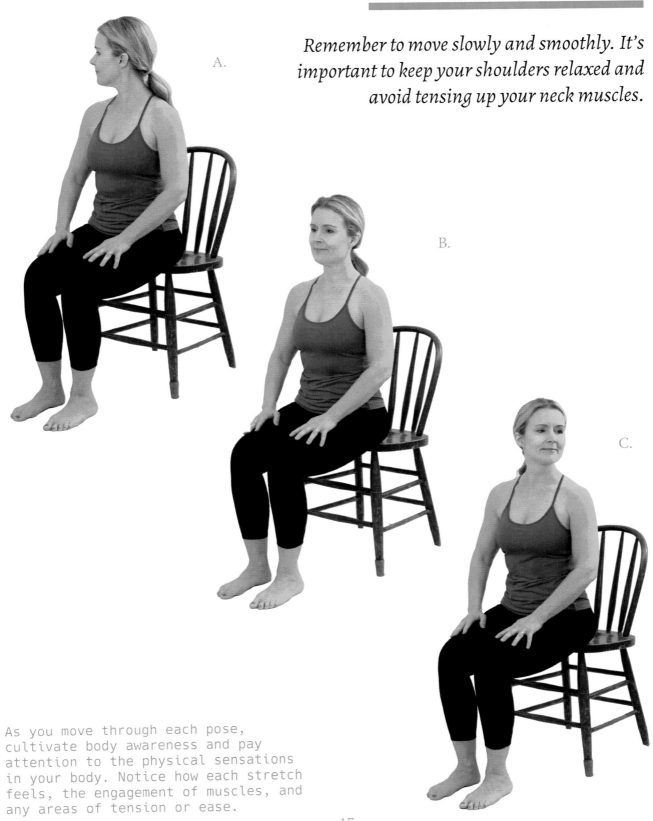

Remember to move slowly and smoothly. It's important to keep your shoulders relaxed and avoid tensing up your neck muscles.

A.

B.

C.

As you move through each pose, cultivate body awareness and pay attention to the physical sensations in your body. Notice how each stretch feels, the engagement of muscles, and any areas of tension or ease.

LATERAL NECK STRETCH

This gentle stretch will help you find relief from tight, aching muscles in your upper back, neck and shoulders.

1. Sitting tall with your core engaged, clasp your right hand beneath your chair.

2. Reach your left arm away from your body and toward the earth.

3. Relax your left ear towards your left shoulder and gently lean to the left.

4. Breathe deeply, keeping your spine long and your shoulders relaxed. You should feel a gentle stretch in the right side of your neck all the way down into your right shoulder.

5. Hold this stretch for 5 breaths, and repeat on the opposite side.

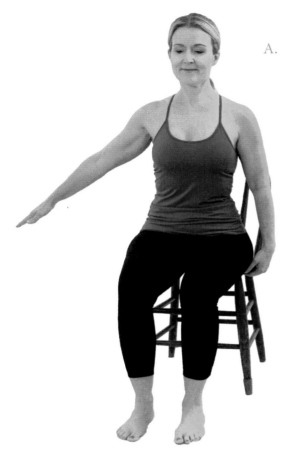

A.

Focus on breathing smoothly and deeply. Make sure to bring your ear towards your shoulder rather than your chin. Keep your spine long and your shoulders down and back.

B.

Let go of expectations and attachments to specific outcomes during your yoga practice. Instead, focus on being fully present and accepting of whatever arises.

19

SHOULDER ROLLS

This movement helps reduce tension and stiffness in the upper back and neck while improving the flexibility and range of motion in your shoulders and upper back.

1. Sit up straight in your chair with your feet flat on the ground and hip width apart.

2. Begin by lifting your shoulders up towards your ears, as if you're trying to touch them to your ears.

3. Next, roll your shoulders backwards, bringing your shoulder blades together.

4. Then roll your shoulders down.

5. Finally, roll your shoulders forward and around, returning to the starting position.

6. Repeat 10x, and then reverse directions. Lift up, forward, down and around.

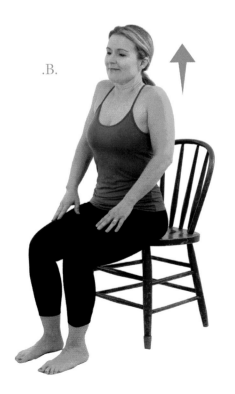

A.

.B.

C.

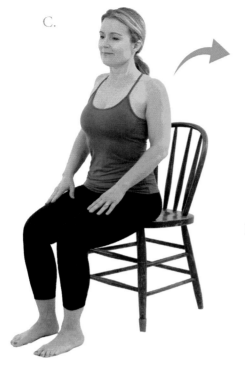

Avoid tensing up your neck or upper back muscles, and focus on keeping your arms relaxed.

D.

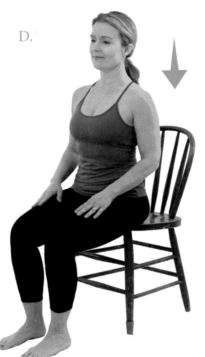

E.

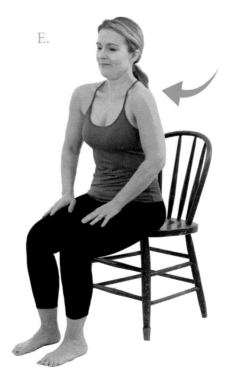

SHOULDER & UPPER BACK STRETCH

This movement can help reduce tension and stiffness in your neck, shoulders and upper back while improving the flexibility and range of motion in your shoulders.

1. Sit up straight in your chair with your feet flat on the ground and hip width apart.

2. Reach your right arm across your body.

3. Use your left arm to gently guide it in across the midline of your body as you reach energetically through your right fingertips.

4. Hold for 5 - 10 breaths and repeat on the opposite side.

To increase this stretch, reach through your fingertips and gently press your right arm into your left using it as added resistance. Keep the tops of your shoulders down and back throughout the stretch.

A.

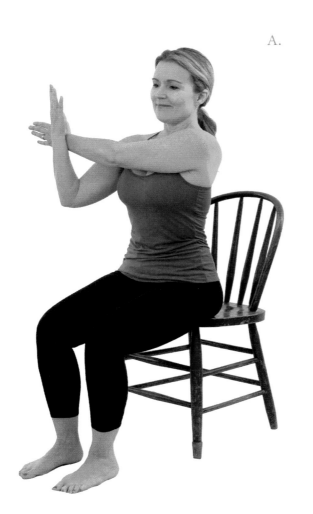

B.

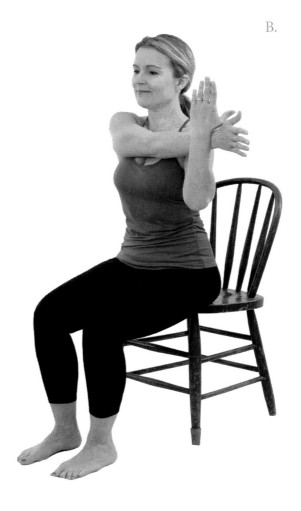

Become the watcher of the thoughts that arise during your practice. Rather than getting caught up in them, simply observe with curiosity and let them pass without judgment.

CAT - COW STRETCH

This pose increases flexibility and mobility in your neck, shoulders, and spine. It also stretches your hips, back, abdomen and chest.

1. Begin by sitting in a comfortable position towards the edge of your chair, with your feet flat on the ground and your hands on your thighs for support.

2. On your inhale, lift your heart, arching your spine while lifting your gaze upwards, creating a cow shape.

3. On your exhale, round your spine, gently drawing your chin towards your chest, creating a "cat" shape with your body.

4. Continue to alternate between the cat and cow positions, moving slowly and smoothly while focusing on your breath.

5. With each inhale, lift through your heart, tilt your pelvis forward lightly. Draw your shoulder blades down your back, gently squeezing them together to support the lift of your chest in a mild backbend.

6. With each exhale, round your spine, curl your tailbone under slightly, and coil your navel back. Gently draw your chin towards your chest, stretching though your lower, mid and upper back.

7. Continue to coordinate this movement with your breath, moving slowly and gently.

8. Repeat for a cycle of 10 - 15 breaths, and then slowly return to an upright position.

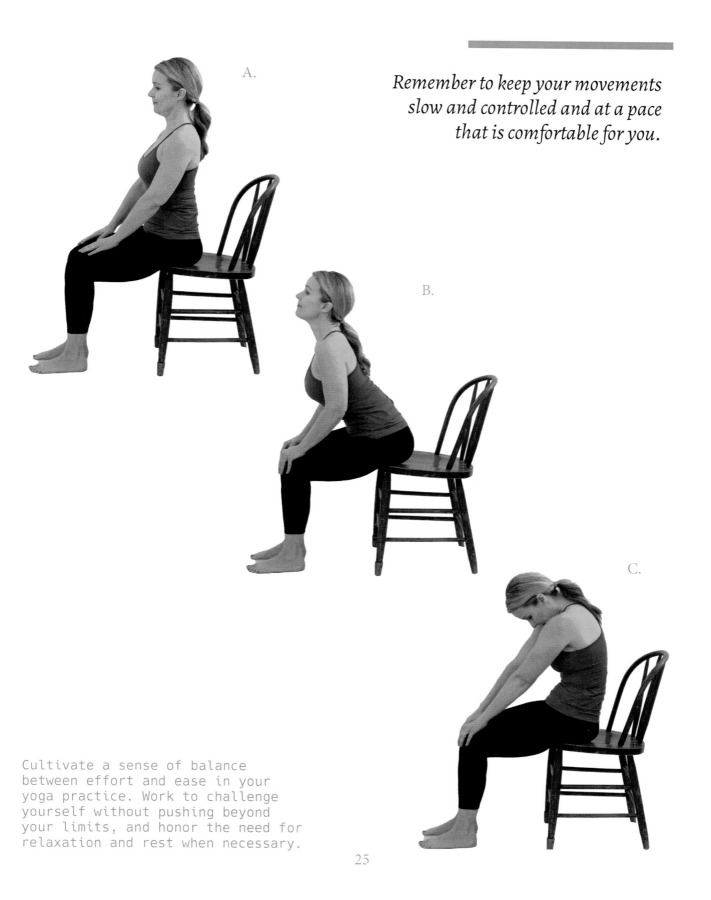

A.

Remember to keep your movements slow and controlled and at a pace that is comfortable for you.

B.

C.

Cultivate a sense of balance between effort and ease in your yoga practice. Work to challenge yourself without pushing beyond your limits, and honor the need for relaxation and rest when necessary.

SIDE STRETCH WITH WRIST PULL

This seated side stretch with wrist pull improves flexibility in your arms, waist and shoulders. It also helps to boost your energy while toning and strengthening your core muscles.

A.

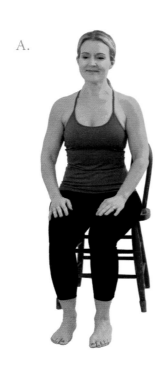

1. Sit up straight with your feet flat on the ground and hip width apart.

2. Inhale, and reach your arms overhead.

3. Exhale as you use your left hand to gently clasp your right wrist reaching up and over to the left, stretching your right side.

4. Continue lifting up and out of both sides of your waist. Keep the weight even in your hips, and lightly lift through your lower belly.

5. Hold this pose for 5 - 10 breaths, focusing on keeping your spine long and your chest open.

6. Release and repeat on the opposite side.

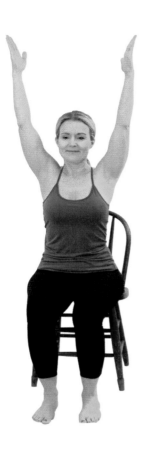

B.

It's important to avoid any sudden movements as you continue breathing deeply, moving slowly and mindfully.

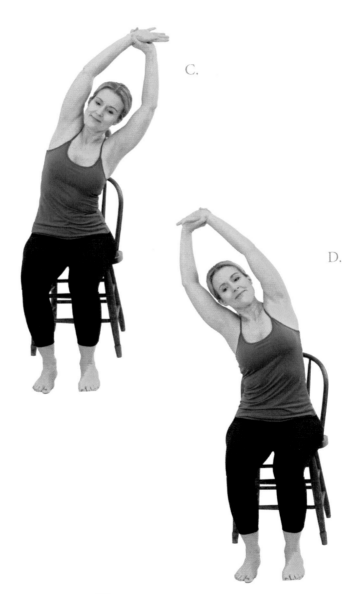

C.

D.

BEHIND THE BACK OPPOSITE ELBOW HOLD

This seated stretch helps to improve your posture while stretching across your chest and shoulders. It's especially helpful for "forward head posture" which happens when the head moves forward and out of alignment with your spine. (Usually associated with jutting your chin forward looking at a cell phone, computer or driving.)

1. Sit up straight with your feet flat on the ground and hip width apart.

2. Reach your arms around behind you and try to clasp opposite forearms or elbows.

3. Keep your shoulders down and back.

4. Hold for 5 - 10 breaths and repeat with your opposite arm on top.

A.

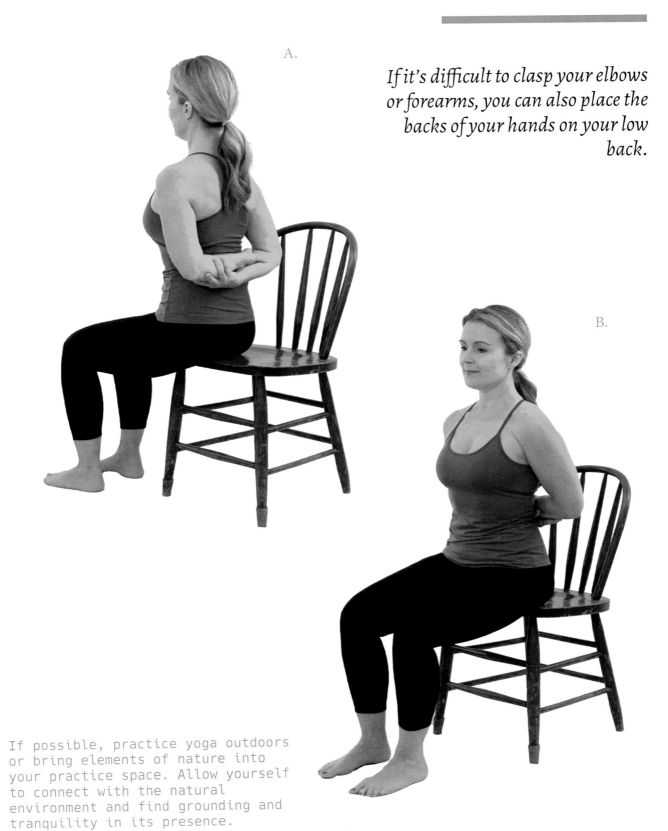

If it's difficult to clasp your elbows or forearms, you can also place the backs of your hands on your low back.

B.

If possible, practice yoga outdoors or bring elements of nature into your practice space. Allow yourself to connect with the natural environment and find grounding and tranquility in its presence.

WRIST ROTATIONS

This exercise helps reduce stiffness and tension while improving the range of motion and flexibility in your wrists and forearms.

1. Sit up straight with your feet flat on the ground and hip width apart.

2. Hold your arms out in front of you with your palms facing down.

3. Make a light fist.

4. Slowly rotate your wrists in a circular motion, making small circles with your wrists.

5. Continue with this movement gradually increasing your range of motion.

6. Repeat 10x and then switch directions.

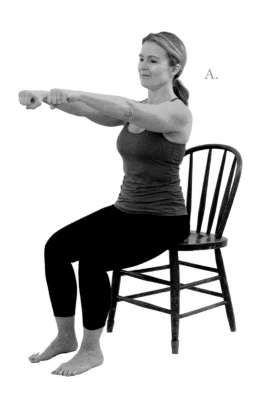

A.

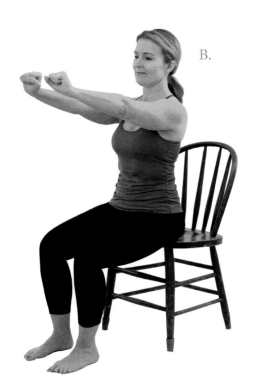

B.

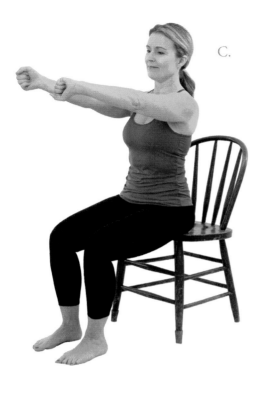

C.

Avoid any sudden movements, moving slowly and smoothly. Do your best to keep your shoulders and arms relaxed as you avoid tensing up your wrists or forearms.

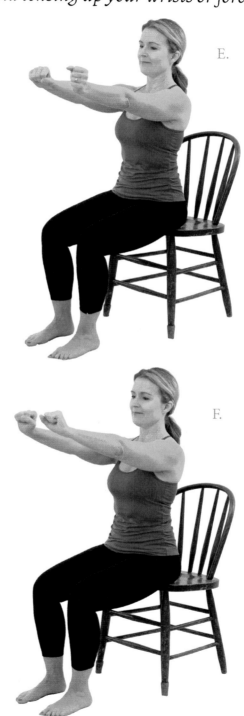

E.

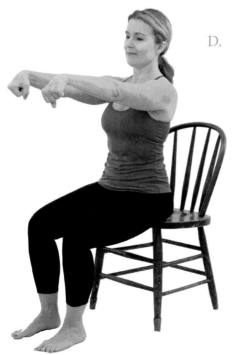

D.

F.

HAND STRETCH

This stretch helps reduce stiffness and tension in your hands and wrists while stretching through your wrists, hands and forearms.

1. Reach your hand out in front of you with your palm facing up and away.

2. Use your opposite hand to gently draw your fingers back towards your body, feeling a stretch in the muscles of your wrist, hand and forearm.

3. Hold for a few breaths, then release and repeat on the opposite side.

A.

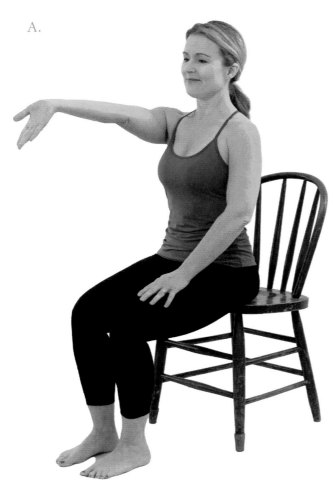

Keep your arm straight as you lengthen through your wrist, gently drawing your fingers back only to comfort level.

B.

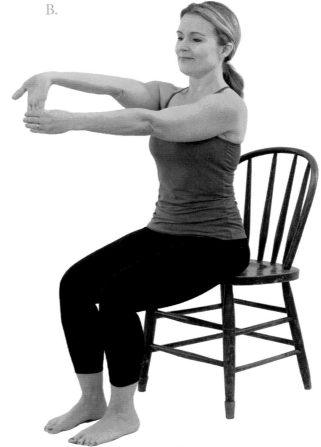

Breathe deeply and smoothly. Use your breath as a tool to anchor your attention in the present moment while cultivating a sense of calm.

DYNAMIC ARM RAISES

This exercise increases circulation in your upper body, stretching through your arms and shoulder joints.

1. Begin by sitting toward the edge of your chair with both feet flat on the ground.

2. Inhale, and sweep your arms forward and up.

3. Exhale, and lower your arms, sweeping down and back.

4. Continue moving at your own pace for 10 cycles, coordinating this movement with your breath.

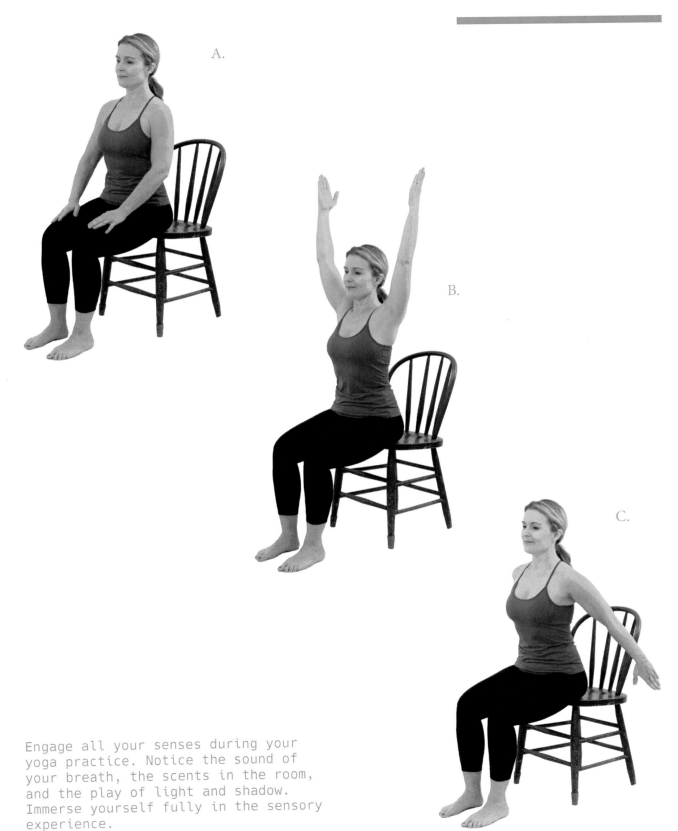

A.

B.

C.

Engage all your senses during your
yoga practice. Notice the sound of
your breath, the scents in the room,
and the play of light and shadow.
Immerse yourself fully in the sensory
experience.

EAGLE POSE

LAYER 1

This pose stretches your shoulders, arms and upper back.

1. Begin by sitting tall with your feet planted firmly on the ground.

2. Lift your chest and engage your core muscles.

3. Reach your arms forward to shoulder height, palms facing upward.

4. Cross your right arm in front of your left for criss-cross arms, palms facing towards you.

5. Gently press your forearms together and lift your arm bones forward and up.

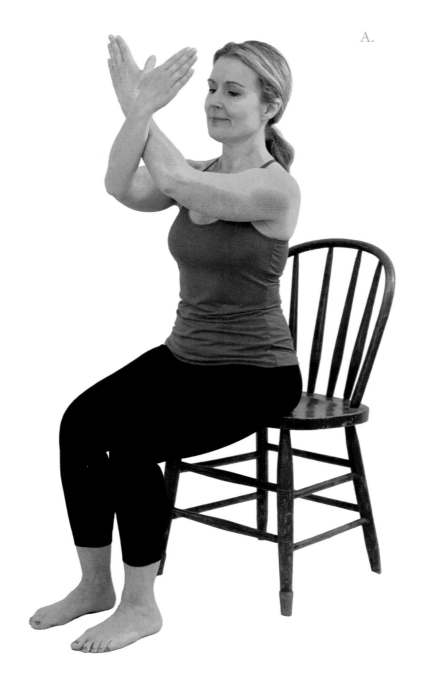

A.

EAGLE POSE

LAYER 2

This pose stretches your shoulders, arms and upper back, and also engages your inner thigh muscles.

6. Stay here, or for an additional stretch, scoop your right arm under your left with the backs of your hands facing each other or press your hands together with your fingertips pointing to the sky.

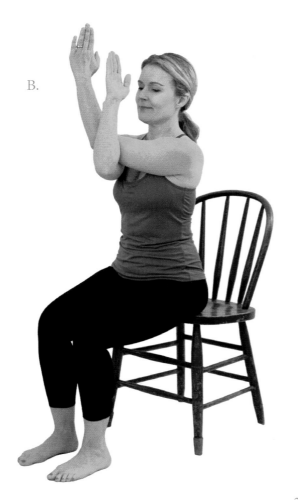

B.

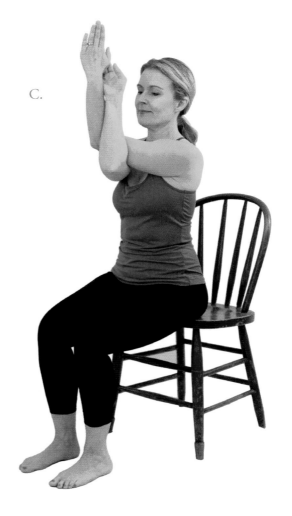

C.

7. Cross your right ankle over your left. Continue here or if space allows, cross your right leg over your left squeezing your thigh bones together.

D..
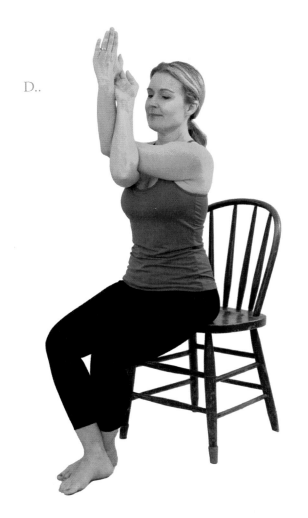

E.
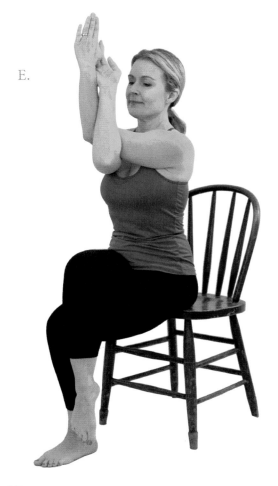

EAGLE POSE

LAYER 3

8. To deepen this stretch, double cross your right foot behind your left leg.

9. Continue to lift your arm bones forward and up feeling a stretch through your shoulders and upper back.

10. Hold this pose for 10 breaths, then slowly return to the starting position and repeat on the opposite side.

Rather than going deeper than is comfortable in this pose, honor your body's feedback and don't push through. Instead, focus on inviting more space and a steady breath.

F.

Keep your core engaged, and make sure to draw your abs in and up. Keep your spine vertical as you lift your ribs up and out of your waist while keeping your shoulders down and back.

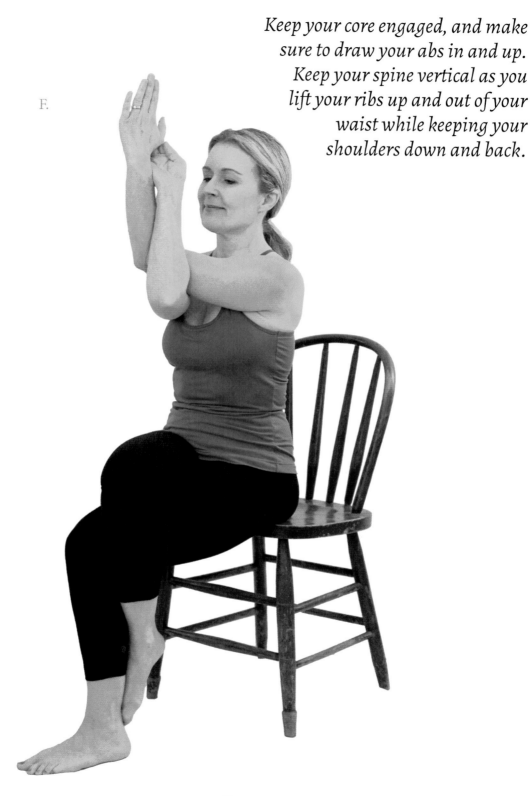

REVERSE PLANK POSITION

This pose opens the front of your body while stretching your shoulders, chest, arms, legs and front ankles.

1. Begin by sitting toward the edge of your chair with both feet flat on the ground.

2. Place your hands to the seat of your chair behind you for support.

3. Inhale, and lift your heart, drawing your shoulder blades down and together to support the lift of your chest.

4. Stay here, or extend both of your legs forward, pressing down through the base of your big toes.

5. Keep your legs strong and active, with your inseams rotating inward slightly.

6. Press your shoulder blades into your back torso to support the lift of your chest for a mild backbend.

7. Hold for 5 - 10 breaths and return to the starting position.

Make sure to breathe smoothly and deeply. Press down through your hands to lift your upper mid back to your sternum and your sternum to the sky. Keep your shoulders down and back and your neck long.

A.

B.

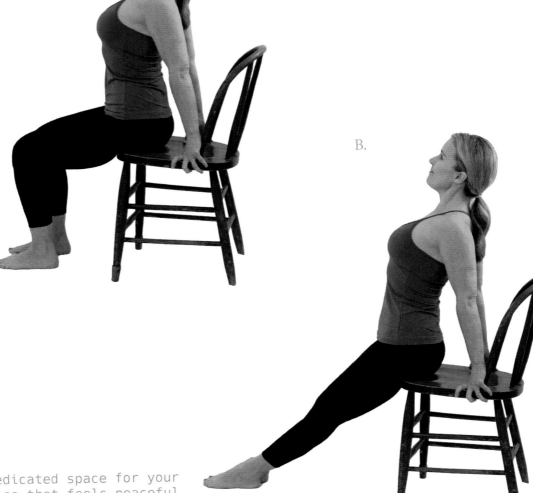

Set up a dedicated space for your yoga practice that feels peaceful and conducive to mindfulness. Clear clutter, bring in elements that inspire tranquility, and create an atmosphere that supports your practice.

SEATED SUN SALUTATIONS

This sequence helps you to feel more focused, improves circulation and digestion, and enhances your breath capacity. It also boosts your muscle tone and creates more flexibility through your spine, arms, legs, hips, shoulders, chest and neck.

1. Adjust to sit toward the front of your chair with your spine long. Sit firmly in your chair, feeling your hips grounded.

2. Keep your feet planted on the ground with your knees over your ankles and your thighs parallel to the ground.

3. With an inhale, sweep your arms overhead reaching only as far as is comfortable for you. Keep your shoulders relaxed, while you lift your ribs up and out of your waist.

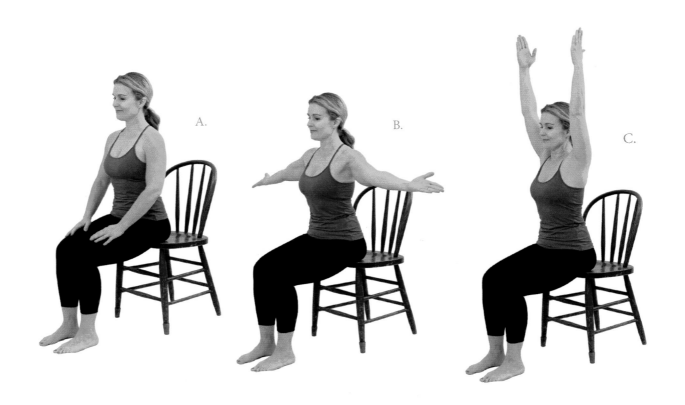

A.

B.

C.

4. Exhale, place your hands to your thighs and gently hinge forward, gliding your hands down your legs. Keep your core engaged as you fold from your hips.

5. With your core engaged, inhale, and come up halfway, lifting your heart to a flat back. With your hands on your legs for support, lengthening your spine and the back of your neck.

6. Exhale, hinge forward from your hip creases, feeling a stretch through the back of your body.

7. Inhale, lift your torso to upright, sweeping your arms overhead.

8. Exhale, release your hands to a prayer position.

9. Continue to coordinate this movement with your breath. Repeat this sequence 5 - 10x.

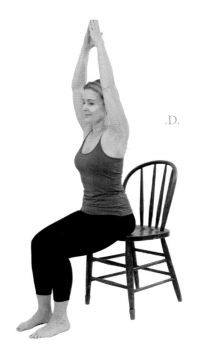 .D.

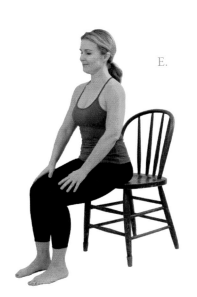 E.

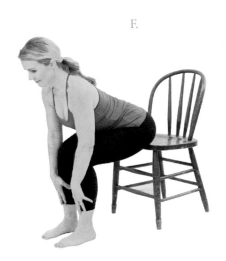 F.

SEATED SUN SALUTATIONS CONTINUED

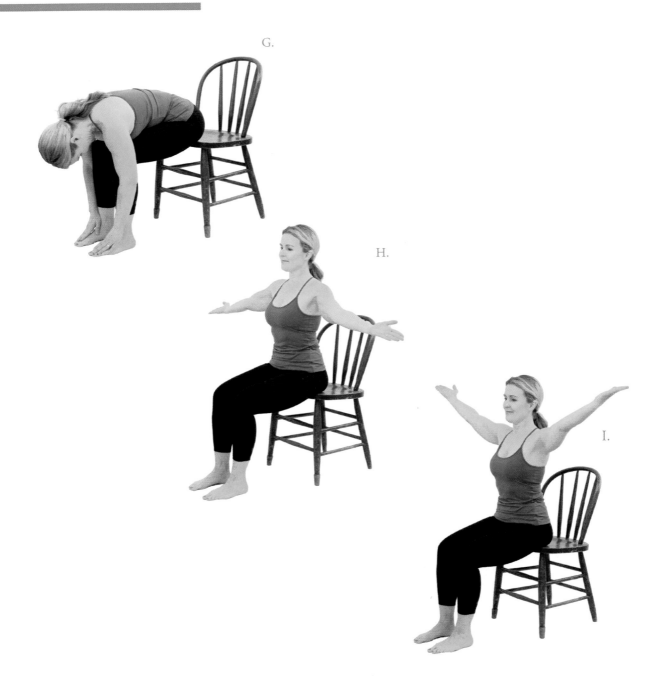

G.

H.

I.

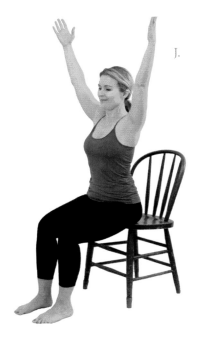

J.

Make sure to keep the majority of your weight in the chair to keep from falling out of your chair. This sequence of movements is a perfect way to start your day, increasing your energy and enhancing your mood. As you practice, continue to breathe smoothly and deeply allowing the flow of the breath and movement to soothe your mind, relax your nervous system, and reduce stress and anxiety.

K.

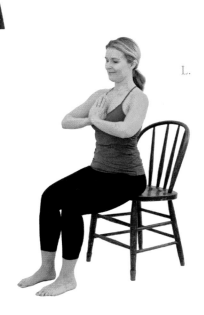

L.

SEATED TWIST

This seated twist pose helps release tension in your back and shoulders while improving flexibility in your spine, chest, shoulders and neck.

1. Sit up straight in your chair with your feet flat on the ground and your arms at your sides.

2. Take a deep breath in. As you exhale, rotate your upper body to the right, placing your left hand to your right leg and your right hand behind you on the chair for support.

3. Maintain your hips facing forward. Rotate from your navel, ribs and chest rather than your hips.

3. Hold this pose for 5 -10 breaths. Focus on keeping your spine straight and your chest open as you continue to lengthen from the base of your spine upwards.

4. To release, exhale to unwind your upper body back to the starting position and repeat on the opposite side.

While practicing this pose, it's important to focus on moving smoothly, slowly, and mindfully.

A.

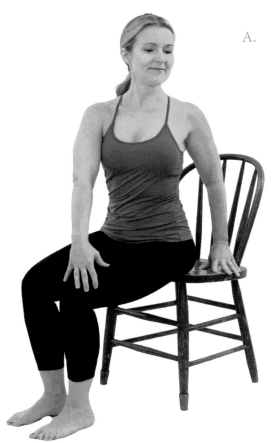

B.

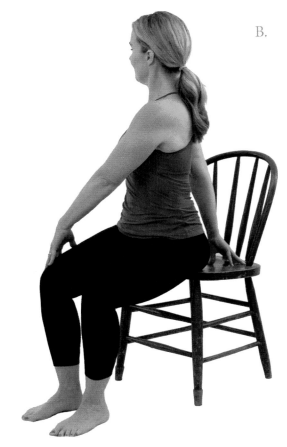

If you need to modify poses or movements to accommodate your body, do so with self-compassion. Honor your body's needs and practice without judgment or comparison to others.

OBLIQUE SIDE CRUNCH

This exercise tones and strengthens your core, targeting your oblique muscles, and tightening the entire side ab wall.

1. Sit tall with your navel back towards your spine.

2. Lightly place your hands behind your head with your elbows wide.

3. Inhale, re-lengthen your spine.

4. Exhale, draw your right elbow toward your right hip.

5. Inhale, lift to upright.

6. Exhale, repeat on the opposite side.

7. Continue for 10 - 15 breaths on each side, coordinating this movement with your breath.

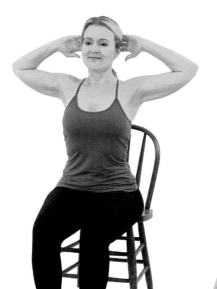

A.

Concentrate on squeezing and contracting through your waist as you lean from side to side, activating your obliques.

B.

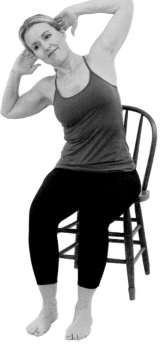

C.

Be aware of your thoughts and emotions as they arise. Observe them without judgment or attachment, allowing them to pass by like clouds in the sky.

ALTERNATE KNEE TUCKS

This exercise directly targets your abs and builds a stronger core while also strengthening your hips flexors and quadriceps.

1. Begin by sitting toward the edge of your chair.

2. Clasp your hands on both sides of the chair for support.

3. Keep your spine straight and your core engaged with your navel back towards your spine. Use your core to stabilize.

4. Extend both of your legs forward.

5. Lean back so your spine is at a 45 degree angle.

6. Inhale. On your exhale, draw your navel back towards your spine, tucking one knee in towards your chest.

A.

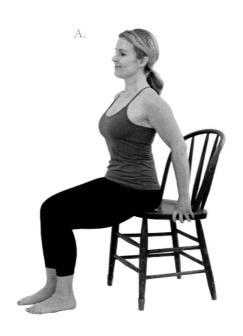

B..

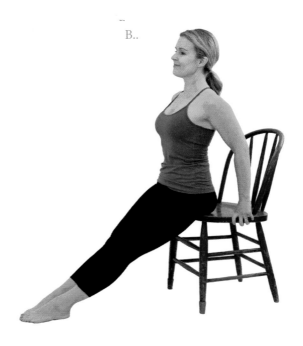

7. Inhale, and lengthen your leg back to starting position.

8. Exhale, and repeat on the opposite side, knee to chest.

Do steps 6-8 for 30 seconds and repeat 2 to 3 rounds if possible, resting when you need to.

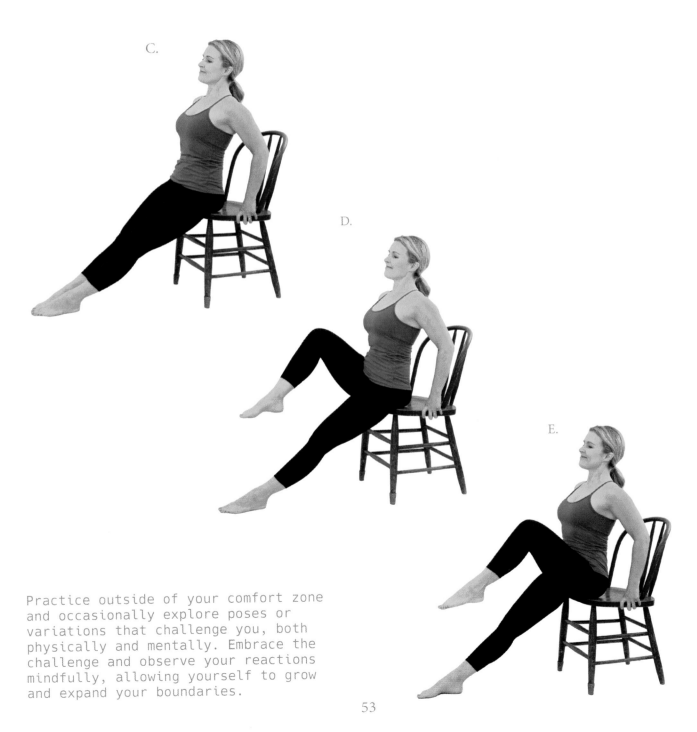

C.

D.

E.

Practice outside of your comfort zone and occasionally explore poses or variations that challenge you, both physically and mentally. Embrace the challenge and observe your reactions mindfully, allowing yourself to grow and expand your boundaries.

FLUTTER KICKS

This exercise works your lower abs along with the hip flexors and quadriceps.

1. Begin by sitting toward the edge of your chair.

2. Clasp your hands on both sides of the chair for support.

3. Keep your spine straight and your core engaged. Draw your navel back towards your spine, using your core to stabilize.

4. Extend both of your legs forward.

5. Lean back so your spine is at a 45 degree angle.

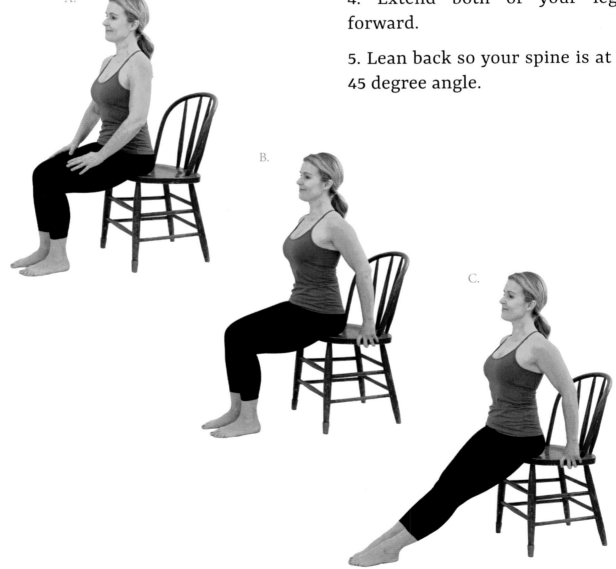

A.

B.

C.

6. Keep your legs straight and strong as you alternate lifting and lowering each leg.

Do step 6 for 30 seconds and repeat 2 to 3 rounds if possible, resting when you need to.

D.

E.

F.

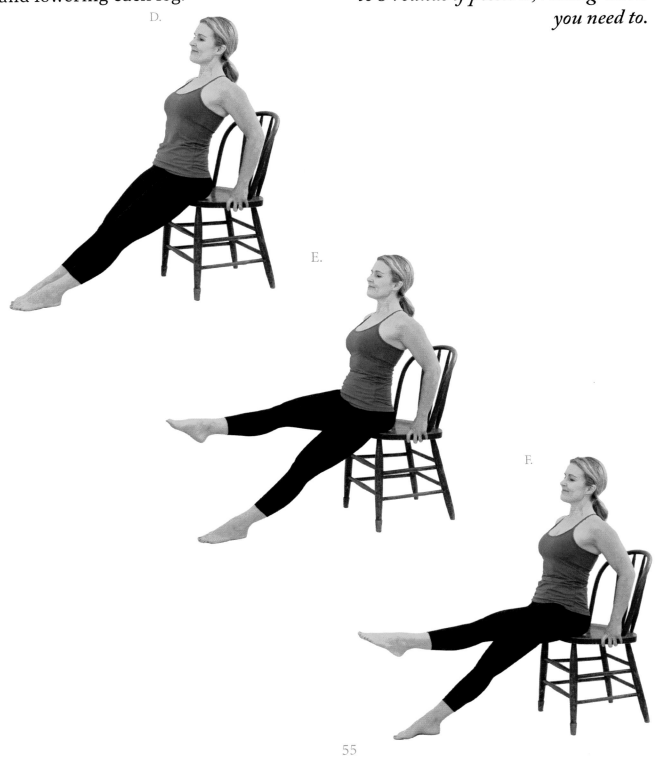

55

KNEE RAISE

This movement strengthens your hip flexors, core and quadriceps.

1. Begin by sitting toward the edge of your chair with both feet flat on the ground.

2. Clasp your hands on the sides of your chair for support.

3. Using your abdominals, focus on lifting your right leg a few inches off the ground. Hold for a few seconds, and then lower back to the starting position.

4. Repeat on the opposite side.

5. Continue with this movement, alternating lifting the right and left leg. Repeat for 10 - 15 cycles.

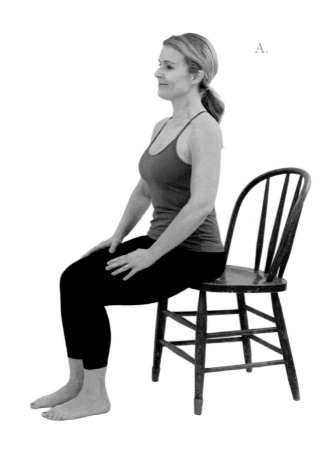

A.

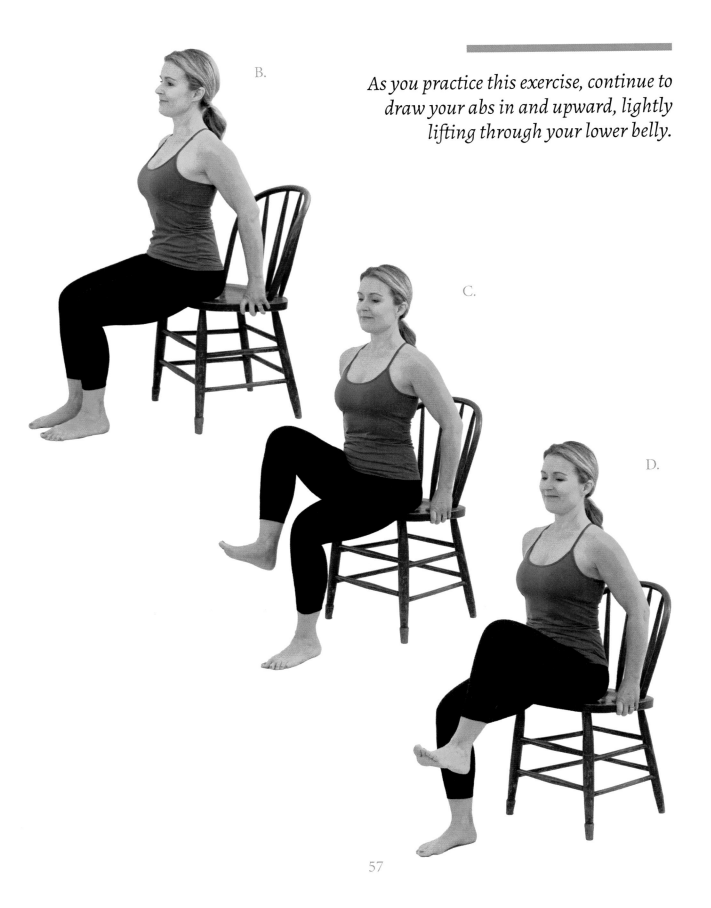

B.

C.

D.

As you practice this exercise, continue to draw your abs in and upward, lightly lifting through your lower belly.

GODDESS POSE

This pose stretches and opens your hips, legs, chest and shoulders while activating your core.

1. Begin by sitting toward the edge of your chair.

2. Step your feet open into a wide stance, turning your toes open slightly, and aligning your knees over your ankles.

3. Lift your chest and engage your core muscles.

4. Raise your arms to shoulder height, with your elbows slightly bent. Keep your shoulders down and relaxed, palms facing upwards.

5. Keep your feet and knees pointing out to the sides, your arms open wide.

6. Hold this pose for 10 breaths, then slowly return to the starting position.

Remember to keep your core engaged and your breath steady as you sit tall, lengthen your tailbone towards the earth, and lightly lift your lower belly.

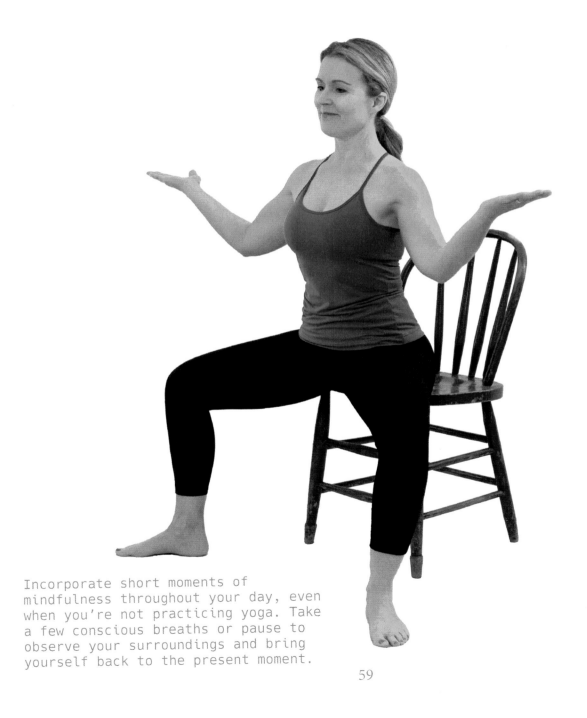

Incorporate short moments of mindfulness throughout your day, even when you're not practicing yoga. Take a few conscious breaths or pause to observe your surroundings and bring yourself back to the present moment.

GODDESS POSE TORSO CIRCLES

This movement stretches your inner thighs, back and abs while activating your core.

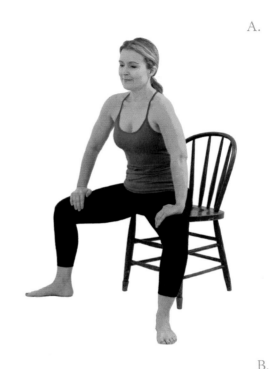

A.

1. Begin by sitting towards the edge of your chair and step your feet into a wide stance with your toes turned open slightly.

2. Place your hands on your thighs, fingers pointing inwards.

3. Use your abs to circle your torso in a clockwise direction feeling this action stretch through the front, back and sides of your core.

4. Continue for 10 cycles and then rotate in the opposite direction.

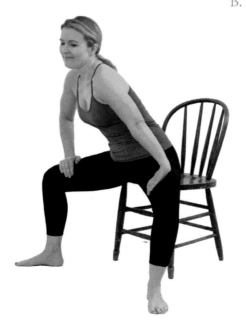

B.

5. When finished, return to upright and step your feet back to center.

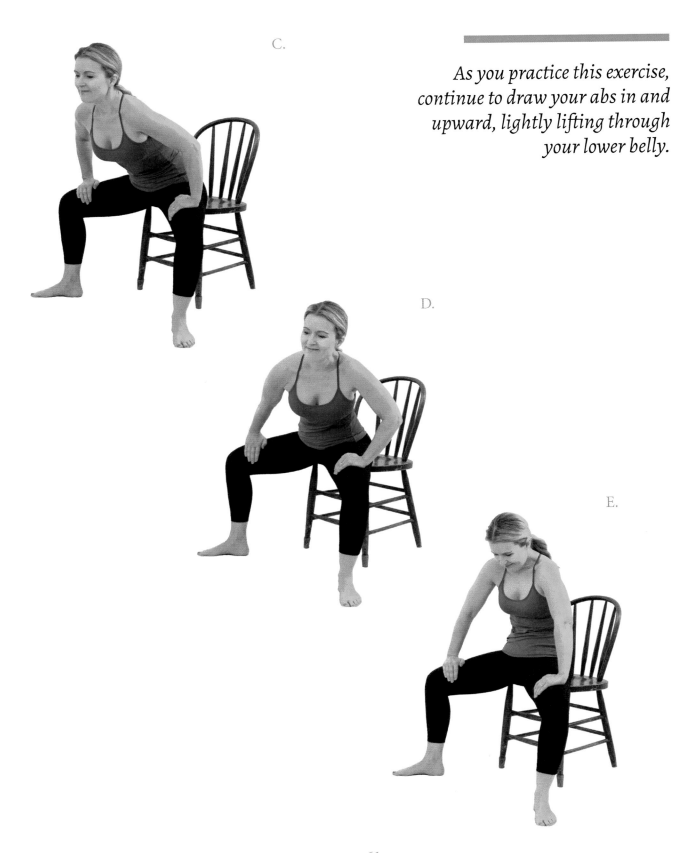

C.

D.

E.

As you practice this exercise, continue to draw your abs in and upward, lightly lifting through your lower belly.

GODDESS DIAGONAL STRETCH

This pose stretches through your inner thighs, spine, shoulders and chest.

1. Begin by sitting towards the edge of your chair and step your feet into a wide stance with your toes turned open slightly.

2. Place your hands on your thighs, fingers pointing inwards.

3. Inhale, and lengthen your spine.

4. Exhale, and stretch your right shoulder towards your left knee.

5. Inhale, lift to upright.

6. Exhale, and repeat on the opposite side.

7. Keep your core engaged and your spine long.

8. Continue alternating right and left for a cycle of 10 breaths.

9. When finished, return to upright and step your feet back to center.

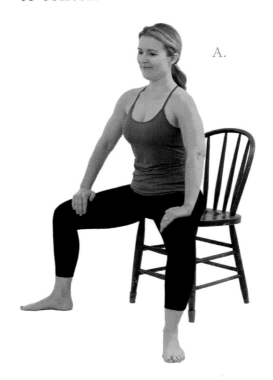

A.

B.

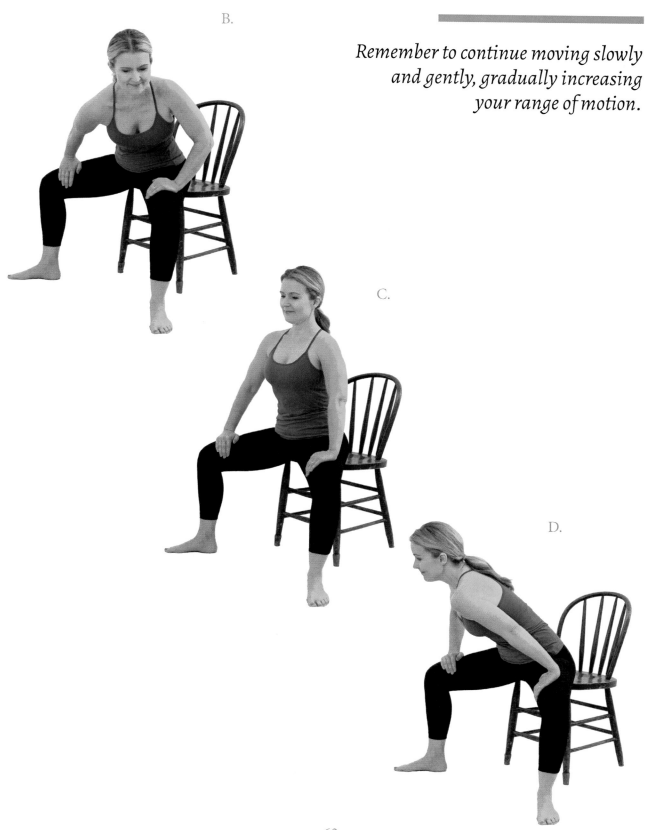

Remember to continue moving slowly and gently, gradually increasing your range of motion.

C.

D.

63

HIP CIRCLES

This movement helps to warm up your hips, release tension, and create more mobility and flexibility in your hip joints.

1. Begin by sitting toward the edge of your chair with both feet flat on the ground.

2. Sitting tall, draw your right knee in towards your chest.

3. With your right hand on your right leg, begin to circle your right leg open in a clockwise direction for an external hip rotation.

4. Repeat 5 - 10 times and then switch directions adding an internal hip rotation, rotating in a counterclockwise direction.

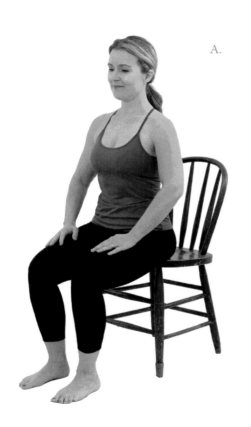

A.

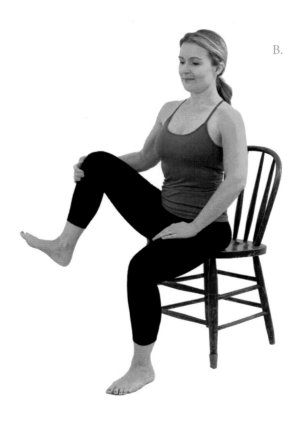

B.

5. Release and repeat on the opposite leg.

Make sure to move slowly and gently, gradually increasing your range of motion.

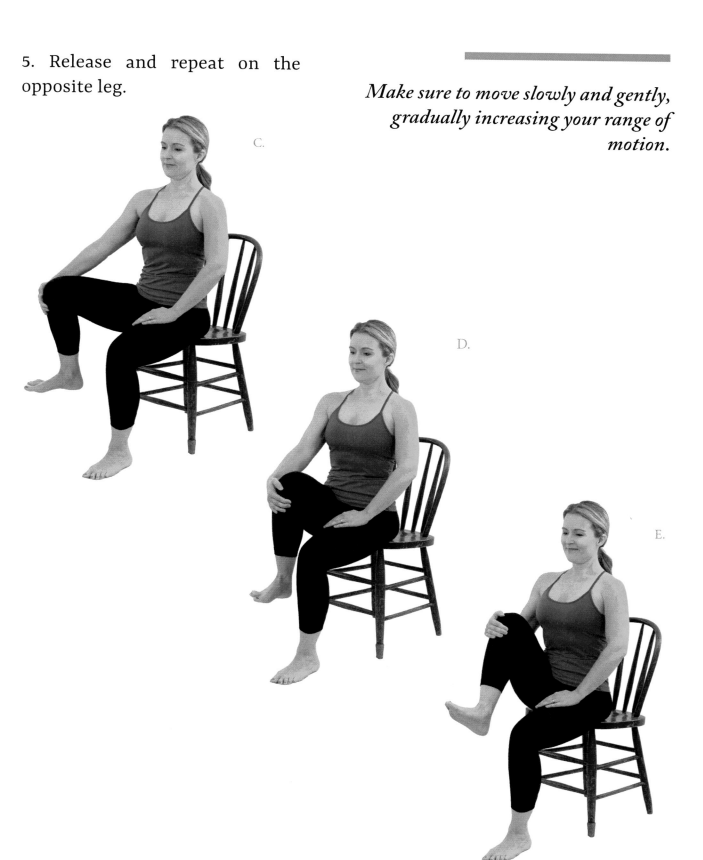

C.

D.

E.

FIGURE FOUR HIP OPENER

This pose is a great hip opener, helping to release tension in your low back, inner thighs, glutes and outer hips.

1. Begin by sitting tall with your feet planted firmly on the ground.

2. Use your hands to draw your right knee in towards your chest.

3. Place your right outer ankle over your left thigh, keeping your right foot flexed and in line with your right knee. Continue sitting tall, and relax your right thigh open.

4. Stay here, or to increase this stretch, clasp your hands to the outer sides of the seat of your chair, and inhale to lengthen your spine.

5. Exhale, and gently fold forward from your hips.

6. Hold for 10 - 15 breaths, and repeat on the opposite side.

A.

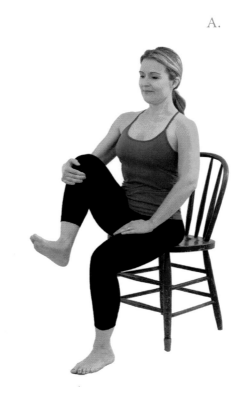

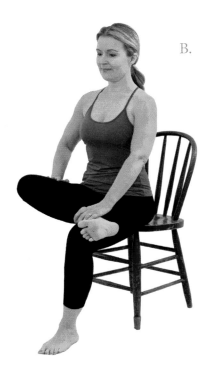

B.

Move slowly and gently, and without forcing. Give your muscles time to relax into this stretch.

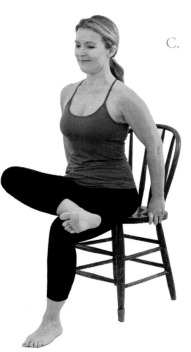

C.

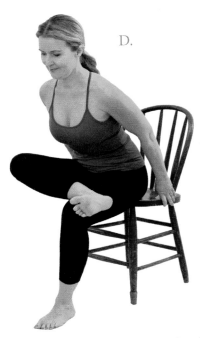

D.

Integrate mindful pauses during your practice. Pause between poses or movements to reconnect with your breath and sensations, and check in with your body and mind.

TREE POSE

This pose stretches your hips, inner thighs, groin muscles, spine, chest, shoulders and arms.

1. Begin by sitting tall with your feet planted firmly on the ground.

2. Use your hands to draw your right knee in towards your chest.

3. Place your right outer ankle over your left thigh, keeping your right foot flexed and in line with your right knee.

4. Place your hands together either in a prayer position or reach your arms overhead.

5. Keep your spine long, lengthen your tailbone towards the earth, and lightly lift through your lower belly.

6. Maintain space and a steady breath. Find a gazing spot to rest your eyes, and feel your mind become calm and focused.

7. Hold this pose for 5 - 10 breaths.

8. To release the pose, use your hands to uncross your leg and slowly lower your right foot back down to the ground. Repeat on the opposite side.

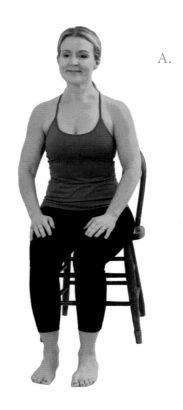

A.

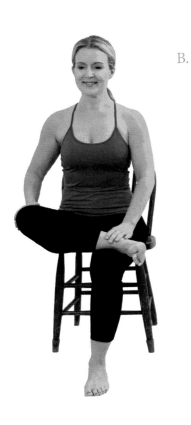

B.

Because we are seated and have removed the element of balance, you can explore going deeper into this pose by settling down through your sitting bones and lifting up through your spine.

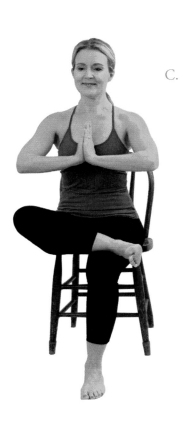

C.

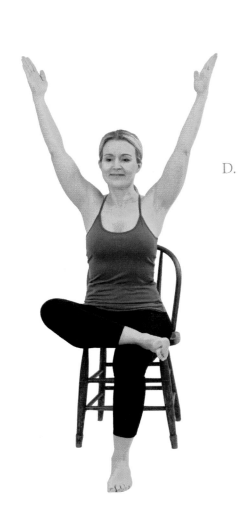

D.

LEG EXTENSIONS

This movement creates more mobility in your knee joints, stretching your hamstrings, calf muscles, and feet.

1. Begin by sitting toward the edge of your chair with both feet flat on the ground.

2. Sitting tall, draw your right knee in towards your chest.

3. Clasp both hands beneath your right leg.

4. Extend your right leg, lengthening through your heel.

5. Bend at your knee, keeping your right foot flexed.

6. Continue with this movement for a cycle of 10 and repeat on the opposite side.

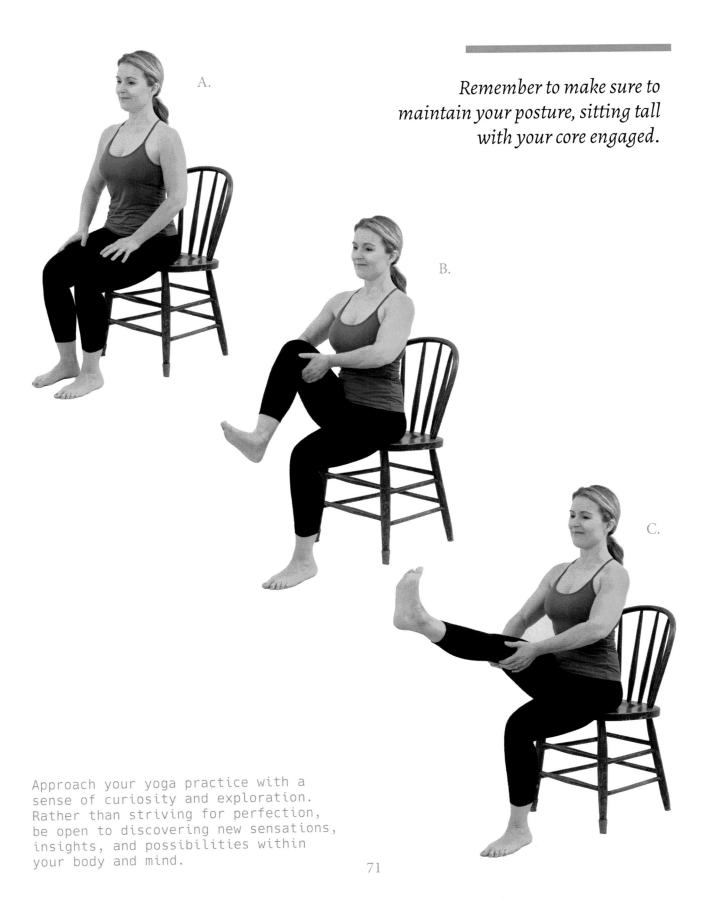

A.

B.

C.

Remember to make sure to maintain your posture, sitting tall with your core engaged.

Approach your yoga practice with a sense of curiosity and exploration. Rather than striving for perfection, be open to discovering new sensations, insights, and possibilities within your body and mind.

71

POINT AND FLEX

This movement helps to stretch and strengthen your feet, ankles, calves and shins.

1. Begin by sitting toward the edge of your chair with both feet flat on the ground.

2. Sitting tall, draw your right knee in towards your chest.

3. Clasp both hands beneath your right leg and extend your right leg straight.

4. Point your toes away, and flex your toes back.

5. Continue with this movement for a cycle of 10, and repeat on the opposite side.

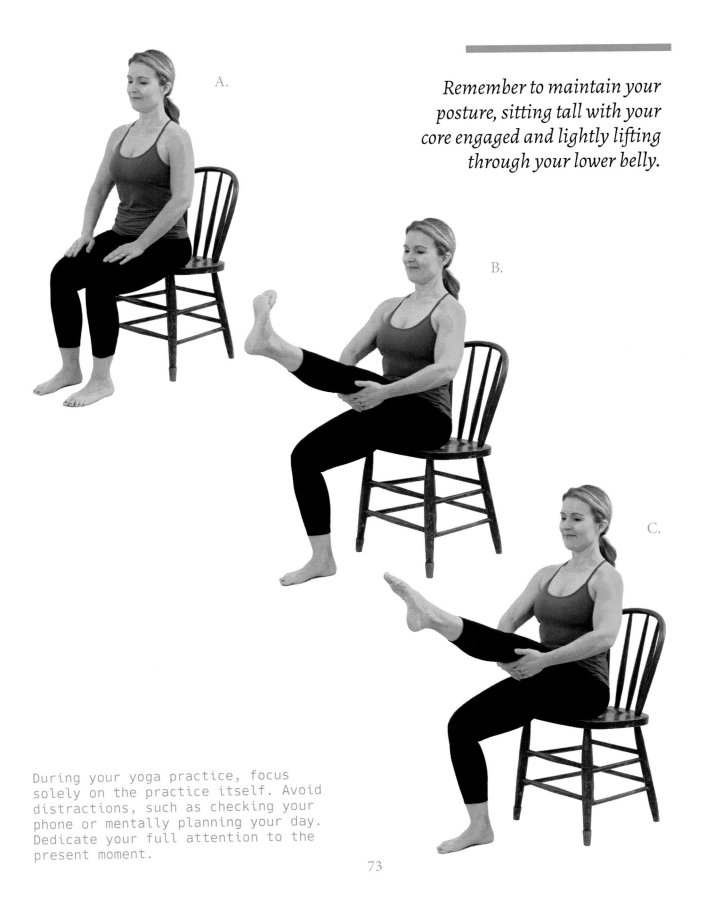

A.

B.

C.

Remember to maintain your posture, sitting tall with your core engaged and lightly lifting through your lower belly.

During your yoga practice, focus solely on the practice itself. Avoid distractions, such as checking your phone or mentally planning your day. Dedicate your full attention to the present moment.

ANKLE ROTATIONS

Ankle rotations create more mobility in the ankle joints, strengthen your shins, and release tension through the tops of your feet, sole and ankle.

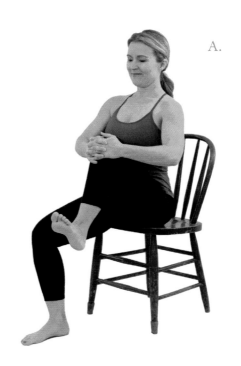

A.

1. Begin by sitting toward the edge of your chair with both feet flat on the ground.

2. Sitting tall, use both hands to draw your right knee in towards your chest.

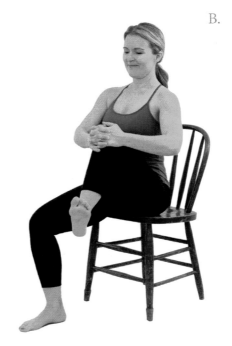

B.

3. Begin to circle your right foot in a clockwise direction 10 times.

4. Repeat rotations in a counterclockwise movement 10 times.

5. Release and repeat on the opposite side.

C.

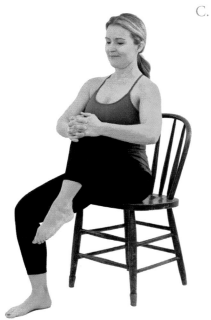

Make sure to move slowly and gently, gradually increasing your range of motion.

D.

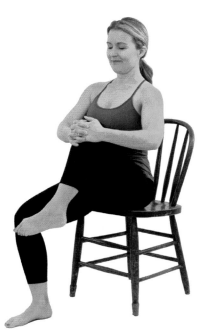

E.

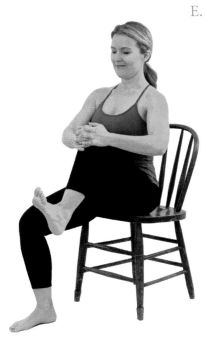

ONE LEGGED SEATED FORWARD BEND

This forward bend variation helps to open and stretch the entire back of your body, including your hips, hamstrings, inner thighs and spine. It also helps to calm your mind and relieve stress.

1. Sitting tall towards the edge of your chair, extend your right leg forward, rooting down through your right heel, flexing through your right foot.

2. Place your hands on your left thigh for support.

3. Inhale, lengthen your spine.

4. Exhale, fold forward from your hip creases. Keep your core engaged and your right leg active by contracting your thigh muscles, and flexing though your right heel.

5. Hold for 10 breaths and repeat on the opposite side.

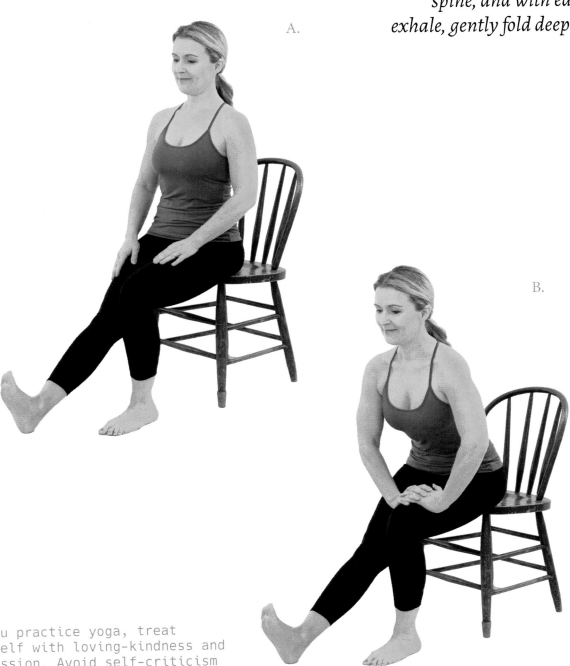

Continue breathing deeply as you hold this stretch. With each inhale, lengthen your spine, and with each exhale, gently fold deeper.

A.

B.

As you practice yoga, treat yourself with loving-kindness and compassion. Avoid self-criticism and offer yourself acceptance in each moment.

LUNGE POSE

Lunge pose helps to stretch and strengthen your legs and improve flexibility in your hips.

1. Begin by sitting a little more right on your chair with your hands on your thighs.

2. Walk your feet over to the right side of your chair.

3. Keep your right thigh on the chair as you extend through your left leg. Lift your left hip off the chair and come onto the ball of your left foot with your left heel raised.

4. Lengthen your tailbone towards the earth while lifting through your lower belly. Keep your front knee over your front ankle.

5. Lift through your chest and engage your core muscles.

6. Inhale and reach your arms overhead, lightly lifting through your lower belly. Reach through your fingertips as you maintain the energy and alignment in your legs.

7. Hold this pose for 5 breaths, then slowly return to center. Repeat on the opposite side.

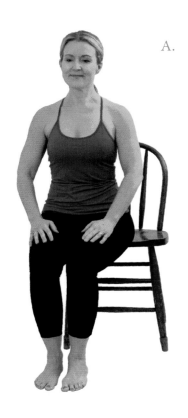

A.

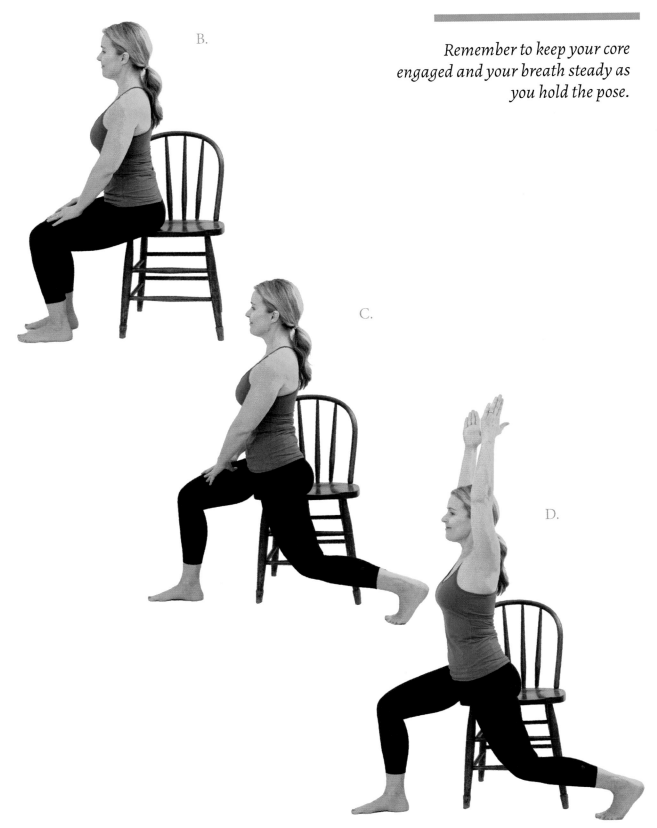

B.

C.

D.

Remember to keep your core engaged and your breath steady as you hold the pose.

WARRIOR 2 POSE

Warrior 2 helps to build strength and improve balance by working your legs, glutes, hips, abs and arms.

1. Begin by sitting toward the edge of your chair with your feet hip width apart and your hands on your thighs.

2. Step your right foot open to the right towards a 90 degree angle. Point your right toes open, and align your right knee over your right ankle.

3. Keep your left foot pointing straight ahead. Stay here, or for more of a challenge, extend through your left leg, and press down through the outer edge of your left foot. Turn your left toes inward at a slight angle.

4. Lift your chest and engage your core muscles.

5. Keeping your shoulders relaxed and your neck long, raise your arms parallel to the earth, and reach out energetically through your fingertips.

6. Gently turn your head to look out over your right hand.

7. Stay firm in your legs by grounding down through both feet, and keeping your front knee aligned over your front ankle.

8. Keep your hips even, with your torso aligned over your hips.

9. Hold this pose for 5 - 10 breaths, then slowly return to the starting position. Repeat on the other side.

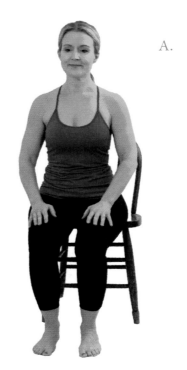

A.

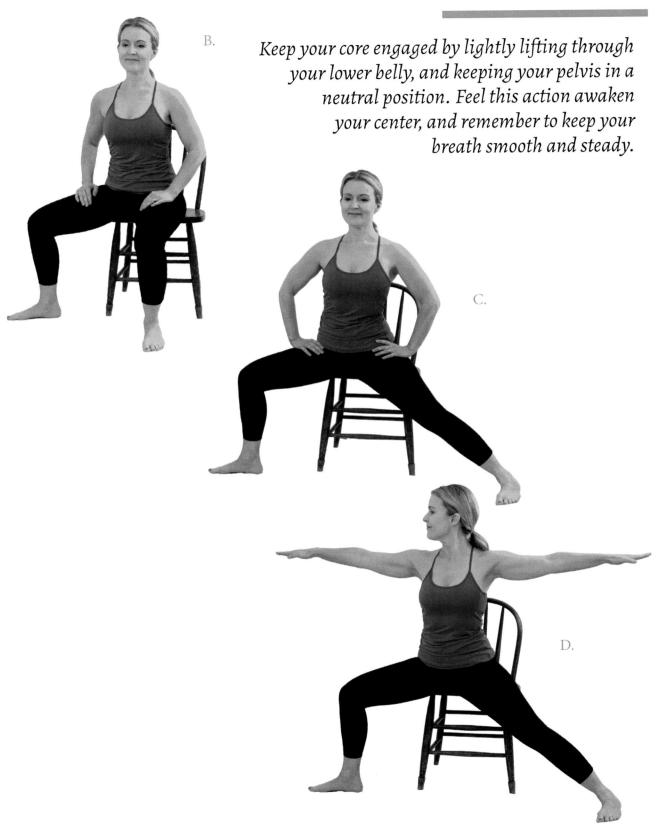

B.

Keep your core engaged by lightly lifting through your lower belly, and keeping your pelvis in a neutral position. Feel this action awaken your center, and remember to keep your breath smooth and steady.

C.

D.

EXTENDED SIDE ANGLE POSE

Extended side angle pose helps to improve flexibility in your hips and spine and strengthen your legs and glutes.

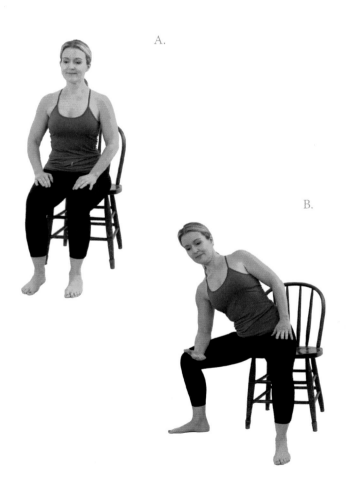

A.

B.

1. Begin by sitting toward the edge of your chair with your feet hip-width apart and your hands on your thighs.

2. Step your right foot open to the right towards a 90 degree angle. Point your right toes open, aligning your right knee over your right ankle.

3. Keep your left foot pointing straight ahead.

4. Engage your core muscles. Inhale, lengthen your spine.

5. Exhale and lean your upper body to the right. Bring your right forearm to your right thigh, and keep your top shoulder open to the sky.

6. Reach your left arm overhead, palm facing downward.

7. For more of a challenge, extend through your left leg, press down through the outer edge of your left foot, and turn your left toes inward at a slight angle.

8. To increase this stretch, gently turn your head to look towards your top arm as you continue to roll your top shoulder open to the sky, broadening across your collarbones.

9. Lengthen your heart away from your navel as you reach energetically through your top arm, lengthening through your left side body.

10. Energize through your legs, by pressing your thigh bones back towards the back of your body, and your sit bones into your front body at equal rate, opening across your hips.

11. Hold this pose for 5 - 10 breaths, then slowly return to the starting position. Repeat on the opposite side.

Remember to keep your core engaged and your breath smooth and steady as you hold this pose.

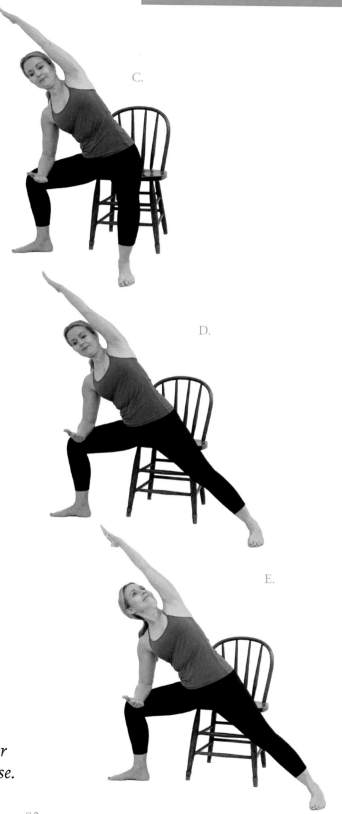

TRIANGLE POSE

Triangle pose activates your core muscles, helping with stability and balance. It's also a great stretch for your spine, hips, legs and shoulders.

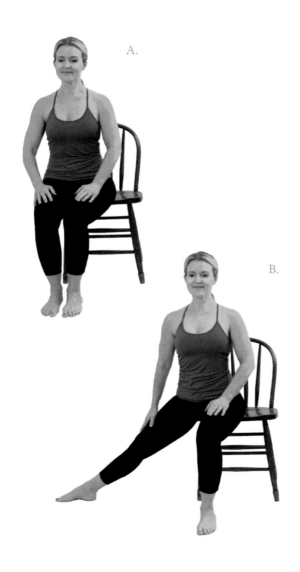

A.

B.

1. Begin by sitting toward the edge of your chair with your feet hip width apart and your hands on your thighs.

2. Adjust your weight to sit a little more towards the right side of your chair.

3. Extend your right leg open to the right, pointing your right toes open, and rooting down through both feet.

4. Inhale, raise your arms like a T, parallel to the earth.

5. Exhale, and with your core engaged, extend and lengthen your upper body out over your right leg.

6. Rest your right hand lightly above or below your right knee.

7. Reach your top arm to the sky.

8. To increase this stretch, gently turn your head to look towards your top arm.

9. Hold this pose for 5 - 10 breaths, then slowly return to the starting position.

10. Repeat on the opposite side.

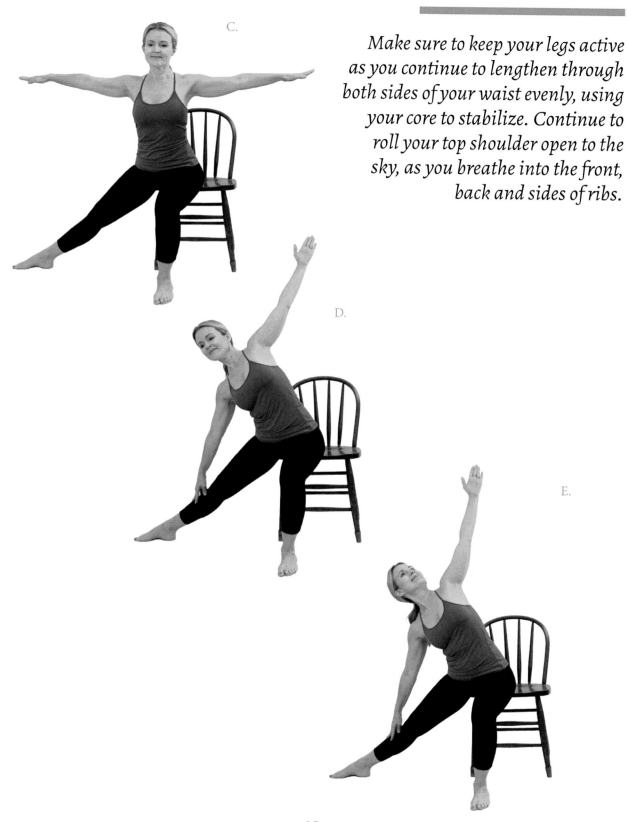

C.

Make sure to keep your legs active as you continue to lengthen through both sides of your waist evenly, using your core to stabilize. Continue to roll your top shoulder open to the sky, as you breathe into the front, back and sides of ribs.

D.

E.

SAVASANA

Savasana, or Corpse Pose is a resting posture performed at the end of your yoga practice. Savasana helps to integrate the benefits of your yoga practice into your body and allows your body and mind to fully relax and rest. While your body is in a relaxed state, your mind is encouraged to let go of stressful thoughts and tension. This deep relaxation helps to reduce stress and anxiety, lower your blood pressure and promote better sleep. It's also an opportunity for reflection. By letting go of external distractions and focusing inward, you can begin to cultivate greater self-awareness and inner peace.

1. Find a comfortable and quiet space to sit in a chair with your feet flat on the ground and your back straight, but not tense.

2. Take a few deep breaths, inhaling through your nose and exhaling through your mouth. Let any tension in your body release as you slowly exhale.

3. Gently close your eyes and bring your attention to your breath. Focus on the sensation of the breath moving in and out of your body.

4. Begin to scan your body from your head down to your toes, noticing any areas of tension or discomfort. As you exhale, imagine that tension melting away, allowing your muscles to fully relax.

5. Feel your breath easy and natural now, breathing in and out through your nose, as you consciously relax your body one area at a time.

6. Start by focusing your attention on your forehead and release any tension held there. Allow your forehead to

Remember, you can practice this relaxation exercise whenever you need a moment of calm and peace throughout the day.

feel smooth and calm and all the tiny muscles in your face soften.

7. Move your attention down to your jaw and allow it to soften and release any tension held there. Release your tongue from the roof of your mouth and the backs of your teeth. Let your teeth be slightly apart and your lips be gently closed.

8. Focus on relaxing through your neck and shoulders, releasing any tension held there. Allow your shoulders to relax down away from your ears.

9. Move your attention down to your arms and hands. Feel your arms release and let your hands be soft and relaxed.

10. Move your attention down to your chest and belly. Allow your breath to flow naturally, without effort, and let your chest and belly expand and contract with each inhale and exhale.

11. Focus on your low back, mid back, and upper back, and release any tension held there. Allow your back to be supported by your chair.

12. Move your attention down to your hips and legs. Allow your legs to relax, and release any fatigue you feel there.

13. Let your feet rest comfortably on the ground, relaxing the soles of your feet, toes and ankles.

14. Take a few more deep breaths, feeling a sense of calm and relaxation throughout your body. Continue relaxing, letting go of any unnecessary effort in your body as you rest.

15. When you are ready, gently open your eyes and take a moment to notice how you feel. Carry this sense of relaxation and calm with you as you go about your day.

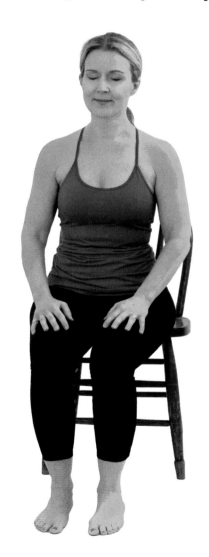

MORNING STRETCH

Start your day off right with a burst of energy and positivity! This gentle morning stretch will help increase flexibility & mobility, improve circulation and reduce stress! So roll out of bed, grab your chair and enjoy a quick morning stretch that will leave you feeling refreshed and ready to tackle your day!

1. Cat/Cow (page 24)

2. Sun Salute (page 44)

3. Shoulder Rolls (page 20)

4. Lateral Neck Stretch (page 18)

5. Side Stretch w/ Wrist Pull (page 26)

6. Dynamic Arm Raises (page 34)

7. Knee Raise (page 56)

8. Goddess Pose Torso Circle (page 60)

9. Hip Circles (page 64)

10. Leg Extension (page 70)

11. Ankle Rotation (page 74)

1.

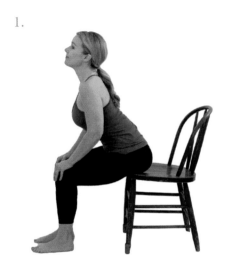

2.

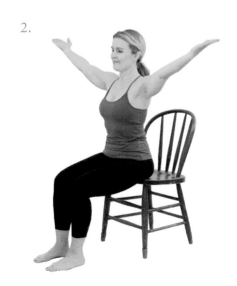

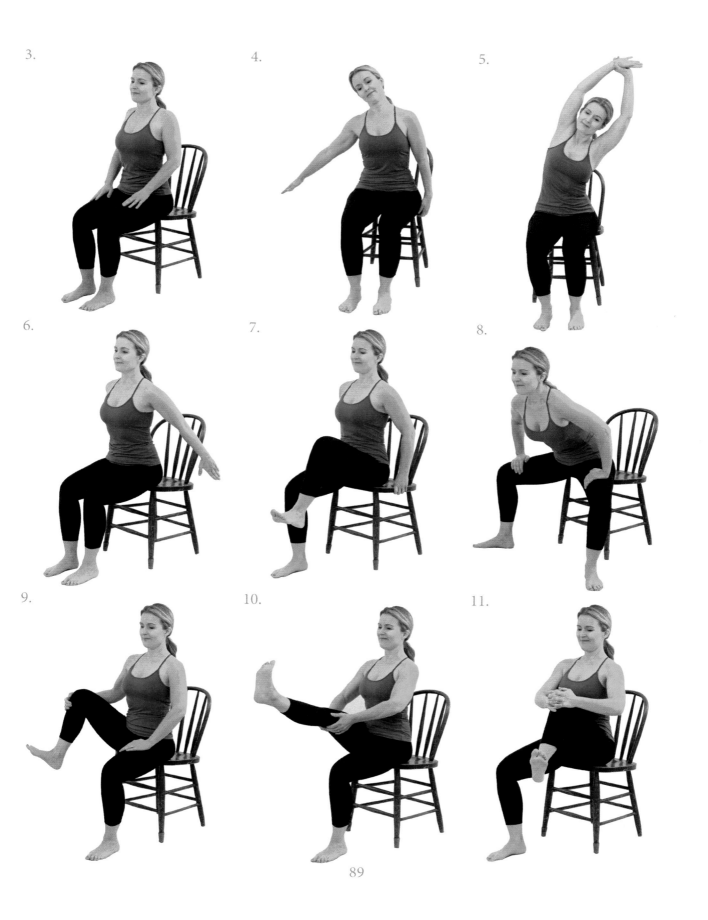

10 MIN. TOTAL BODY STRETCH

Rejuvenate from head to toe with this total body stretch! Use this quick routine a few times a week to improve joint mobility and circulation, increase your range of motion and release tension in your whole body.

1. Shoulder Rolls (page 20)

2. Lateral Neck Stretch (page 18)

3. Side Stretch with Wrist Pull (page 26)

4. Hand Stretch (page 32)

5. Hip Circles (page 64)

6. Figure 4 Stretch (page 66)

7. Leg Extensions (page 70)

8. Ankle Rotations (page 74)

9. One Legged Forward Bend (page 76)

10. Cat-Cow Stretch (page 24)

11. Seated Twist (page 48)

12. Savasana (page 86)

1.

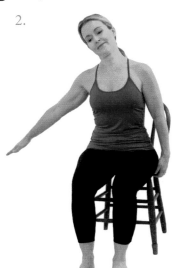

2.

3.

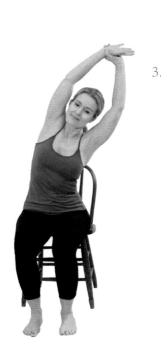

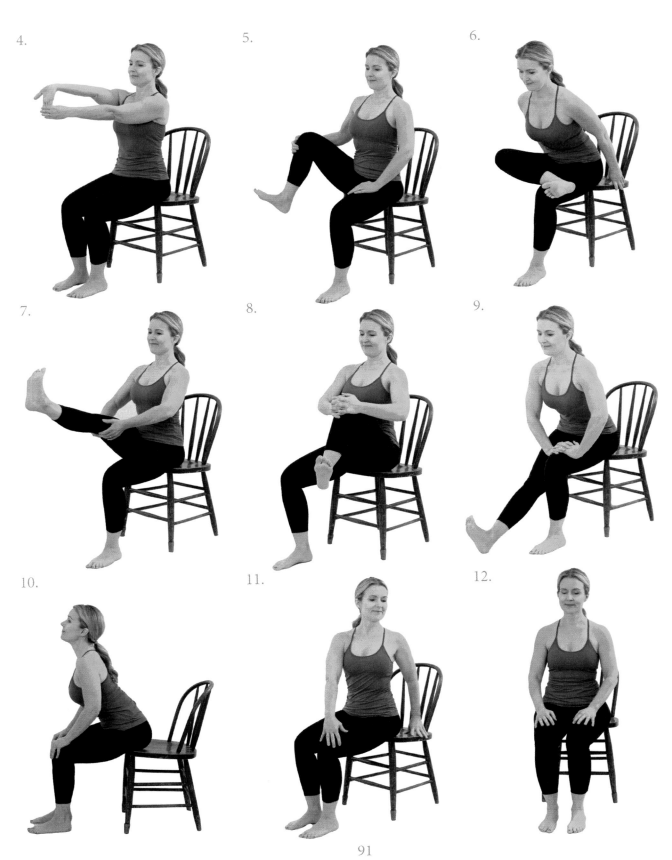

AB FOCUSED ROUTINE

A strong core can not only improve your posture and help alleviate lower back pain, but it can also increase stability and balance. These core focused moves engage and challenge multiple muscles in different ways, leading to a more functional core. The best part is you can stay right in your chair!

1. Cat/Cow (page 24)

2. Oblique Side Crunch (page 50)

3. Knee Raise (page 56)

4. Alternate Knee Tucks (page 52)

5. Flutter Kick (page 54)

6. Goddess Diagonal Stretch (page 62)

7. Seated Twist (page 48)

1.　　　　　　　2.　　　　　　　3.

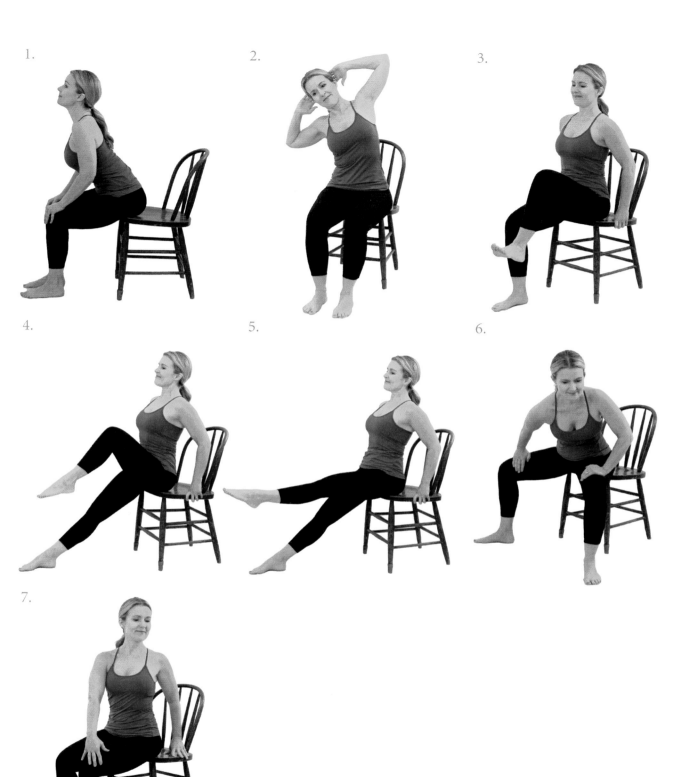

4.　　　　　　　5.　　　　　　　6.

7.

HIP & BACK RELIEF

Create more mobility, release tension and reduce pain in your hips and lower back with this seated routine designed to stretch your hips, hamstrings, low back and more!

1. Cat/Cow (page 24)

2. Side Stretch w/ Wrist Pull (page 26)

3. Hip Circles (page 64)

4. Figure Four Hip Opener (page 66)

5. Leg Extension (page 70)

6. One Leg Seated Forward Bend (page 76)

7. Behind the Back Opp. Elbow (page 28)

8. Reverse Plank (page 42)

9. Cat/Cow (page 24)

10. Tree Pose (page 68)

11. Goddess Pose Torso Circle (page 60)

12. Goddess Pose Diagonal Stretch (page 62)

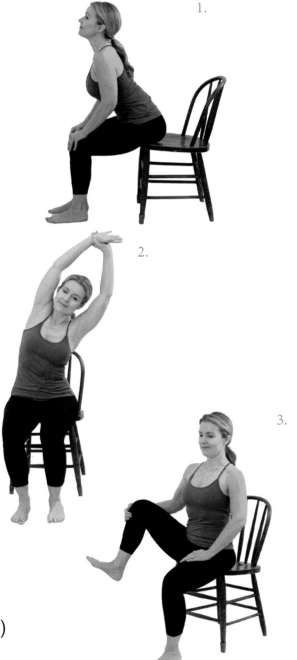

1.

2.

3.

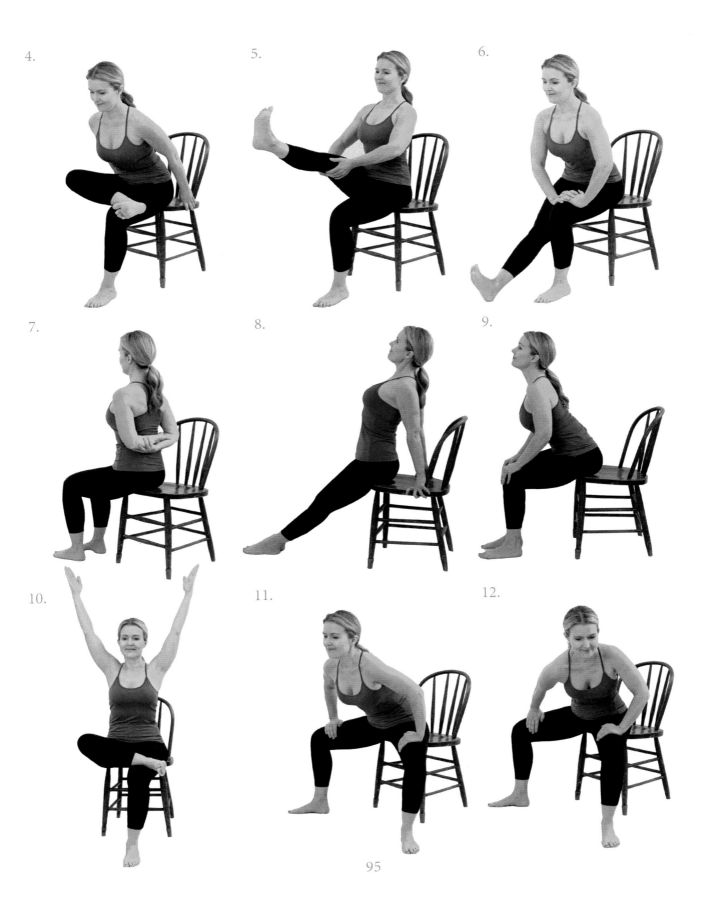

STRENGTH ROUTINE

Tone and strengthen with this quick but very beneficial yoga routine to tone your legs and open your hips, along with upper body stretches designed to increase mobility in your spine, arms, shoulders and chest.

1. Dynamic Arm Raises (page 34)

2. Knee Raises (page 56)

3. Leg Extension (page 70)

4. Hip Circles (page 64)

5. Eagle Pose (page 36)

6. Lunge Pose (page 78)

7. Triangle Pose (page 84)

8. Warrior 2 Pose (page 80)

9. Extended Side Angle Pose (page 82)

10. Goddess Pose (page 58)

11. Goddess Pose Diagonal Stretch (page 62)

12. Tree Pose (page 68)

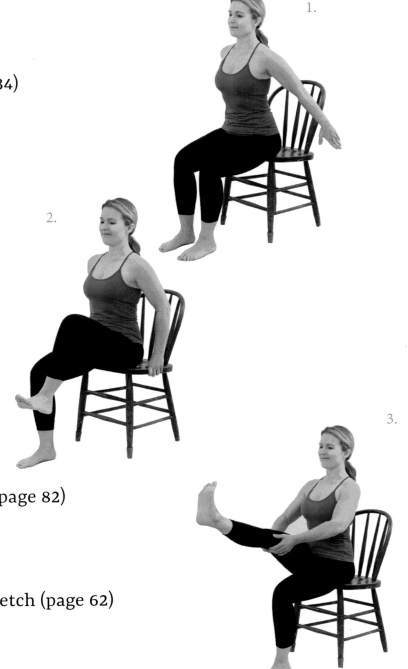

4.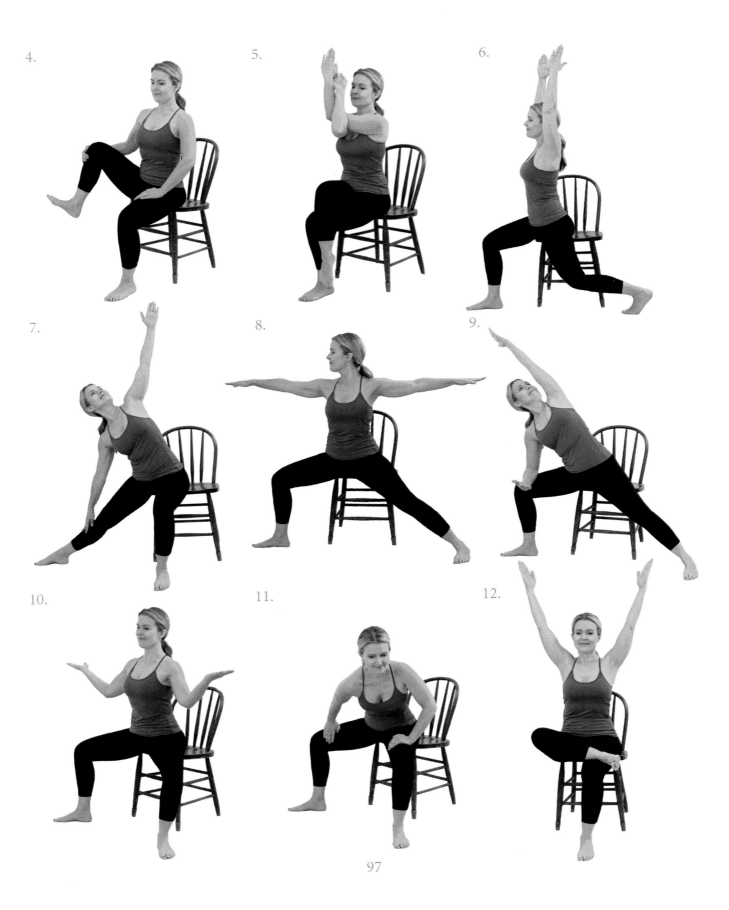

5.

6.

7.

8.

9.

10.

11.

12.

97

UPPER BODY TENSION RELIEF

Relax and refresh with this gentle routine, releasing tension in your upper body while improving range of motion in your joints. Increase flexibility in your neck, chest, shoulders, arms and back, keeping your muscles and joints flexible so you can move through your day without pain... especially helpful for those who sit at a desk all day!

1. Shoulder Shrugs (page 14)

2. Neck Rotations (page 16)

3. Lateral Neck Stretch (page 18)

4. Shoulder Rolls (page 20)

5. Shoulder & Upper Back Stretch (page 22)

6. Cat-Cow Stretch (page 24)

7. Side Stretch with Wrist Pull (page 26)

8. Behind the Back Opposite Elbow Hold (page 28)

9. Wrist Rotations (page 30)

10. Hand Stretch (page 32)

11. Sun Salutations (page 44)

12. Seated Twist (page 48)

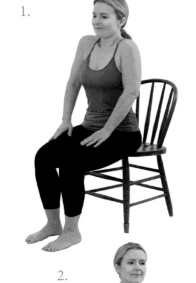

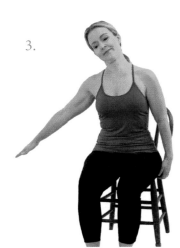

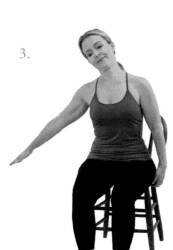

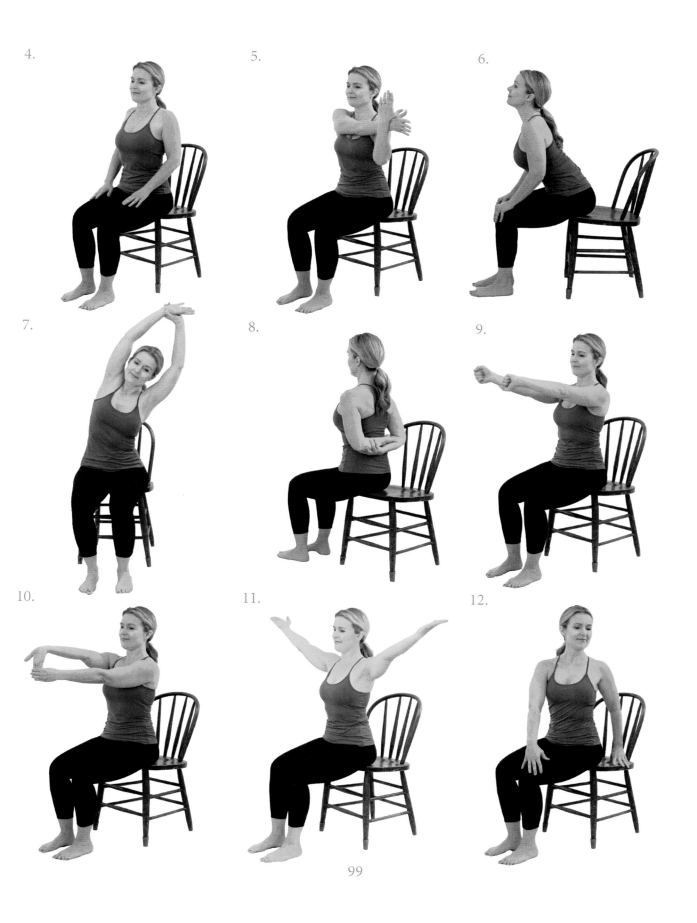

4.

5.

6.

7.

8.

9.

10.

11.

12.

BEDTIME RELAXATION ROUTINE

Release tension and clear your mind with this gentle yoga practice designed to target those tight spots where tension tends to get stuck and starts to build up in your body, (especially areas like your neck, shoulders and upper back!)

1. Three Part breath (page 12)

2. Neck Rotation (page 16)

3. Shoulder shrugs (page 14)

4. Lateral Neck Stretch (page 18)

5. Shoulder Rolls (page 20)

6. Shoulder & Upper Back Stretch (page 22)

7. One Legged Forward bend (page 67)

8. Ankle Rotations (page 74)

9. Cat-Cow Stretch (page 24)

10. Seated Twist (page 48)

11. Savasana (page 86)

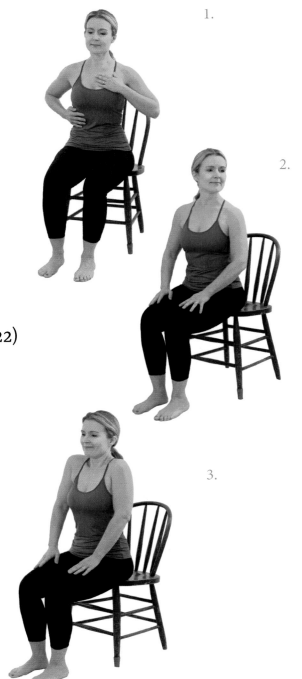

1.

2.

3.

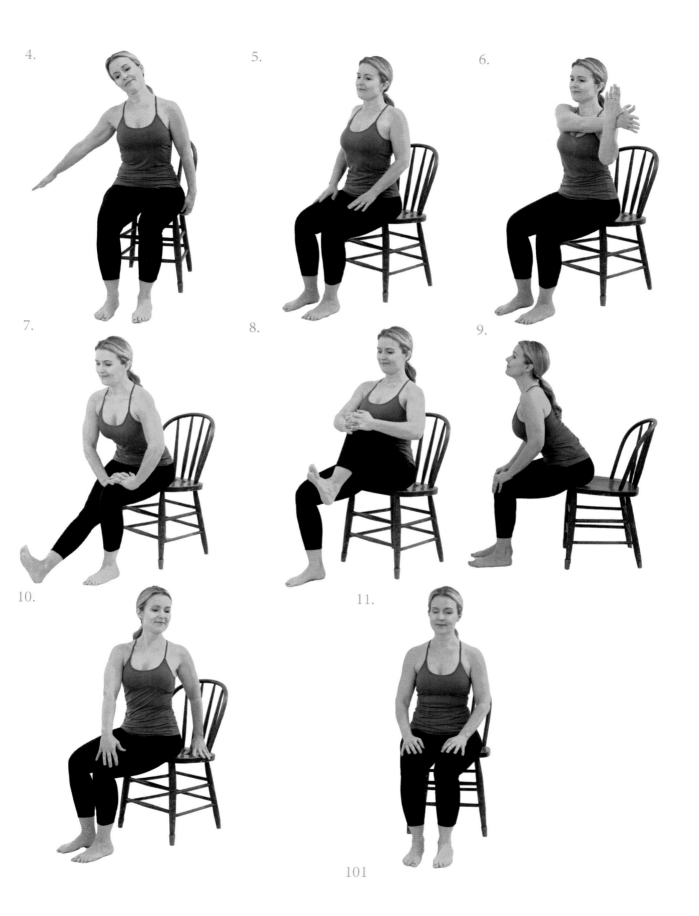

4.

5.

6.

7.

8.

9.

10.

11.

THE END

I hope this yoga practice allows you to feel more relaxed, enthused and confident as you begin your chair yoga journey! Remember to start slowly and gently. Everyone's practice will look a little different and each day will be different. Focus on listening to your body and just simply do your best in each moment. Remember it's a yoga practice and not a yoga "get it done". The joy is in the journey and I can't wait to see where your journey takes you!

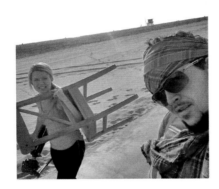

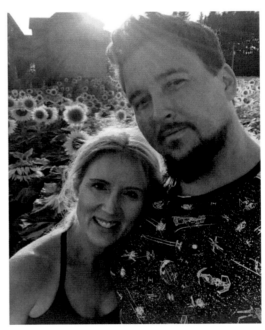

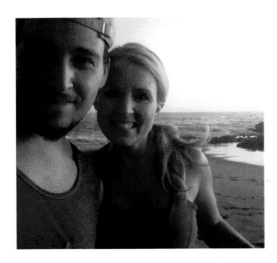

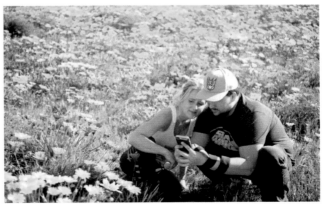

All photography
and design by:
David Starr

And remember your "Happy Yoga"
smile. - Sarah Starr

THE END...

NO IT'S JUST THE BEGINNING!

If you'd like more support on your yoga journey, Happy Yoga On Demand has our entire catalog of over 200 yoga videos that you can stream anywhere, anytime.

WWW.HAPPYYOGAONDEMAND.COM

For our entire catalog of Happy Yoga DVDs visit:

WWW.HAPPYYOGA.TV

Made in the USA
Middletown, DE
06 June 2025

76655501R00058